LOVE YOURSELF, HEAL YOUR LIFE
Workbook

LOVE YOURSELF, HEAL YOUR LIFE Workbook

LOUISE L. HAY

EDEN GROVE EDITIONS

LOVE YOURSELF, HEAL YOUR LIFE WORKBOOK
by Louise L. Hay

Copyright © 1990 by Louise L. Hay

ISBN 1 870845 06 4

Original U.S. Publication by Hay House, Inc.,
Santa Monica, California, U.S.A.

This edition published in Great Britain, 1990 by
Eden Grove Editions
8 The Arena
Mollison Avenue
Enfield
Middlesex EN3 7NJ

The author of this book does not dispense medical advice or prescribe the use of any technique as a form of treatment for physical or medical problems without the advice of a physician, either directly or indirectly. The intent of the author is only to offer information of a general nature to help you in your quest for physical fitness and good health. In the event you use any of the information in this book for yourself, the author and the publisher assume no responsibility for your actions.

Distributed in Great Britain by Airlift Book Company
Printed in Great Britain by The Guernsey Press Co. Ltd, Guernsey, Channel Islands

DEDICATION

W*orkbook* is such a strong word, and many of us feel that hard work is exactly what we must do in order to eradicate old, embedded thought patterns. I don't believe that making inner changes has to be "work," or difficult or painful either. I believe that it can be an adventure.

So, I would like to dedicate this book to the adventurer in *you*. You are on a treasure hunt. Each old negative pattern that you discover is only something to be examined and released. Beneath each pattern is a storehouse of treasure within.

Seek your own gold. Create your own good health. Fill your life with love. Find your own freedom. You are worthy. You do deserve. I will help you.

You are on a pathway to inner enlightenment. As you free yourself, you help to heal the planet.

PART I

INTRODUCTION

BASIC TECHNIQUES

"I am willing to change."

*T*his is a book about change. I know, you want everybody and every-thing else to change. Your mother, father, boss, friend, sister, lover, landlord, neighbor, minister, or government official must change so that your life can be perfect. It doesn't work that way. If you want change in your life, then you are the one who must do the changing. When you change, then all the other people in your world will change in relation to you.

Are you willing to change?

If you are willing, then together we can create the life you say you want. All you have to do is change some thoughts and release some beliefs. Sounds simple? It is. However, it is not always easy. We will explore some of the things you may believe in different areas of your life. If you have positive beliefs, then I urge you to keep them and expand upon them. And if we find negative beliefs, then I will help you let them go.

My life is a good example of what can happen when you change your thinking. I went from being a battered and abused child who grew up in poverty, with little self-esteem and many problems, to a well-known woman who is able to help others. I no longer live in pain and suffering. I have created a wonderful life for myself. You can do it, too.

I encourage you to be gentle with yourself as you embark on the exercises in this workbook. Change can be difficult, or it can be easy. Acknowledge every effort that you make. Know that there may be a transitional period between your old and new belief systems. You may vacillate between former behavior and thinking patterns. Do not be discouraged. Be loving with yourself in the way you would be to a dear friend. Give yourself every encouragement as you go through this new experience.

You will get the quickest results if you can be consistent with the exercises in this book. And yet, even if you can only do one exercise per month, it will still be helpful. Do what you can. The exercises will give you new information about yourself. You will be able to make new choices. Every new choice you make is like planting a seed in your new mental garden. The seeds may take time to germinate and grow. Remember, when you plant a seed, you do not produce an instant apple tree. Similarly, you may not always get instant results from doing this work.

I advise you to use this workbook in sections. Try to do a segment of your life at a time. Really examine your feelings as you do each exercise. Read through the book once. Allow thoughts and memories to come up. Then go back and do all the exercises.

Do the exercises even if you have no problems in that area. You may be surprised at what comes up. Do the exercises several times if it is an area of difficulty for you. Create exercises of your own.

Sometimes it is good to have a box of tissues nearby. Give yourself permission to explore the past and cry if necessary. Tears are the river of life and are very cleansing.

I would like to review the basic beliefs that support my philosophy. You may remember them from *You Can Heal Your Life*.

WHAT I BELIEVE

Life is very simple. What we give out, we get back. I believe that all of us are responsible for every experience in our lives, the best and the worst. Every thought we think is creating our future. Each one of us creates our experiences by the thoughts we think and the words we speak.

Beliefs are ideas and thoughts that we accept as truth. What we think about ourselves and the world becomes true for us. What we choose to believe can expand and enrich our world. Each day can be an exciting, joyous, hopeful experience, or a sorrowful, limiting, and painful one. Two people living in the same world, with the same set of circumstances, can experience life so differently. What can transport us from one world to another? I am convinced that it is our beliefs that do so. When we are willing to change our primary belief structures, then we may experience a true change in our lives.

Whatever your beliefs may be about yourself and the world, remember that they are only thoughts, and thoughts can be changed. You may not agree with some of the ideas that I am about to explore. Some of them may be unfamiliar and frightening. Do not worry. Only those ideas that are right for you will become part of you. You may think that some of the techniques are too simple or foolish and could not possibly work for you. I am only asking you to try them.

Our subconscious mind accepts whatever we choose to believe. The Universal Power never judges or criticizes us. It only accepts us at our own value. If you accept a limiting belief, then it will become the truth for you. If you believe that you are too short, too fat, too thin, too tall, too smart, not smart enough, too rich, too poor, or incapable of forming relationships, then those beliefs will become true for you.

Remember that we are dealing with thoughts, and thoughts can be changed. We have unlimited choices about what we can think, and the point of power is always in the present moment.

What are you thinking in the present moment? Is it positive or negative? Do you want this thought to be creating your future?

When we were children, we learned about ourselves and about life from the reactions of the adults around us. Therefore, most of us have ideas about who we are that we do not own, and many rules about how life ought to be lived. If you lived with people who were unhappy, frightened, guilty, or angry, then you learned a lot of negative things about yourself and your world.

When we grow up, we have a tendency to recreate the emotional environment of our early home life. We also tend to recreate in our personal relationships, those we had with our mother and father. If we were highly criticized as children, then we will seek out those in our adult life who will duplicate this behavior. If we were praised, loved, and encouraged as children, then we will recreate this behavior.

I do not encourage you to blame your parents. We are all victims of victims, and they could not teach you something that they did not know. If your mother or father did not know how to love themselves, it would have been impossible for them to teach you how to love yourself. They were coping as best they could with the information they had. Think for a minute about how they were raised. If you want to understand your parents more, I suggest that you ask them about their childhoods.

Listen to not only *what* they are telling you, but notice what happens to them *while* they are speaking. What is their body language like? Can they make eye contact with you? Look into their eyes and see if you can find their inner child. You may only see it for a split second, but it may reveal some valuable information.

I believe that we choose our parents. I believe that we have decided to incarnate on this earth in a particular time and space. We have come here to learn specific lessons that will advance us on our spiritual, evolutionary pathway. I believe that we choose our sex, color, and country, and then we search for the particular set of parents who will enhance our spiritual work in this lifetime.

All that we are ever dealing with is a thought, and a thought can be changed. No matter what the problem is, your experiences are outer effects of inner thoughts. Even self-hatred is a thought you have about yourself. This thought produces a feeling, and you buy into that feeling. However, if you don't have the thought, you won't have the feeling. Thoughts can be changed. Change the thought, and the feeling must go.

The past has no power over us. It does not matter how long we have been in a negative pattern. We can be free in this moment.

Believe it or not, we do choose our thoughts. We may habitually think the same thought over and over so that it does not seem as if we are choosing the thought. But we did make the original choice. We can refuse to think certain thoughts. How often have you refused to think a positive thought about yourself? You can also refuse to think a negative thought about yourself.

The innermost belief for everyone that I have worked with is always, "I am not good enough!" Everyone that I know or have worked with is suffering from self-hatred or guilt to one degree or another. "I am not good enough, I don't do enough, or I don't deserve this," are common complaints. But for whom are you not good enough? And by whose standards?

I find that resentment, criticism, guilt, and fear cause the most problems in ourselves and our lives. These feelings come from blaming others and not taking responsibility for our own experiences. If we are all responsible for everything in our lives, then there is no one to blame. Whatever is happening "out there" is only a mirror of our own inner thinking.

I do not condone other people's poor behavior, but it is our belief system that attracts this behavior. There is some thought in you that attracts people who exhibit poor behavior. If you find that people are constantly abusing or mistreating you, then this is your pattern. When you change the thought that attracts this behavior, it will stop.

We can change our attitude toward the past. It is over and done, and cannot be changed. Yet we *can* change our thoughts about the past. How foolish for us to punish ourselves in the present moment because someone hurt us long ago.

If we choose to believe that we are helpless victims and that all is hopeless, then the universe will support us in that belief. Our worst opinions of ourselves will be confirmed.

If we choose to believe that we are responsible for our experiences, the good and the so-called bad, then we have the opportunity to outgrow the effects of the past. We can change. We can be free.

The road to freedom is through the doorway to forgiveness. We may not know how to forgive, and we may not want to forgive; but if we are *willing* to forgive, we may begin the healing process. It is imperative for our own healing that *we* release the past and forgive everyone.

This does not mean that I condone poor behavior. I want to encourage the process of setting *you* free. Forgiveness means giving up, letting go. We understand our own pain so well. Yet, it is hard for most of us to understand someone's pain who treated us badly. That person we need to forgive was also in pain. And they were only mirroring what *we* believed about ourselves. They were doing the best they could given the knowledge, understanding, and awareness they possessed at the time.

When people come to me with a problem—I don't care what it is—poor health, lack of money, unfulfilling relationships, or stifled creativity—there is only one thing that I ever work on, and that is *loving the self.*

I find that when we really love, accept, and approve of ourselves exactly as we are, everything in life flows. Self-approval and self-acceptance here and now are the keys to positive changes in every area of our lives.

Loving the self, to me, means to never, ever criticize ourselves for anything. Criticism locks us into the very pattern we are trying to change.

Try approving of yourself and see what happens. You've been criticizing yourself for years. Has it worked?

WORKBOOK TERMINOLOGY

Affirmations

We will be using affirmations throughout this book. Affirmations are any statements that we make—either positive or negative. Too often we think in negative affirmations. Negative affirmations only create more of what we don't want. Saying, "I hate this old car," will get us nowhere. Declaring,

"I bless my old car and release it with love. I now accept and deserve a beautiful, new car," will open the channels in our consciousness to create that.

Make positive statements about how you want your life to be. One important point is: *Always make your statements in the PRESENT TENSE*, such as "I am" or "I have." Your subconscious mind is such an obedient servant that if you declare in the future tense, "I want," or "I will have," then that is where it will always stay—just out of your reach in the future

Dr. Bernie Siegel, bestselling author of *Love, Medicine, & Miracles*, says that "affirmations are not a denial of the present, but a hope for the future. As you allow them to permeate your consciousness, they will become more and more believable until eventually they may become real for you."

Mirror Work

Mirror work is another valuable tool. Mirrors reflect the feelings we have about ourselves. They clearly show us the areas that need to be changed if we want a joyous, fulfilling life.

I ask people to look in their own eyes and say something positive about themselves every time they pass a mirror. The most powerful way to do affirmations is to look in the mirror and say them out loud. You are immediately aware of the resistance and can move through it quicker.

Keep a hand mirror near you as you read this book. Use a larger mirror for some of the deeper exercises.

Visualization

Visualization is the process of using the imagination to achieve a desired result. Put most simply, you see what you want to happen, before it actually does happen.

For example, if what you want is a new place to live, picture a house or an apartment that you want, being as specific as possible. Then see it as if it were already true. Affirm that you deserve it. See your new home with you in it, going about your daily routine. Imagine as clearly as you can, knowing that there is no wrong way to visualize. Practice your visualization frequently, turning all results over to the Universal Mind, and asking for your highest good. Combined with positive affirmations, visualization is a most powerful tool.

Deservability

Sometimes, we refuse to put any effort into creating a good life for ourselves because we believe that we don't deserve it. The belief that we are not deserving may come from our early childhood experiences. Maybe the belief came from our early toilet training. Perhaps we were told that we could not have what we wanted if we did not eat all of our food, clean our room, or put our toys away. We could be buying into another person's concept or opinion that has nothing to do with our own reality.

Deserving has nothing to do with having good. It is our unwillingness to accept that gets in the way. Allow yourself to accept good, whether you think you deserve it or not.

EXERCISE: *Deservability*

Answer the following questions as best you can. They will help you under-stand the power of deservability.

1. What do you want that you are not having?

Be clear and specific about it.

_____

_____

_____

_____

2. What were the laws/rules in your home about deserving?

What did they tell you? "You don't deserve." Or "You deserve a good smack." Did your parents feel deserving? Did you always have to earn in order to deserve? Did earning work for you? Were things taken away from you when you did something wrong?

_____

_____

_____

_____

3. Do you feel that you deserve?

What is the image that comes up? "Later, when I earn it?" "I have to work for it first." Are you good enough? Will you ever be good enough?

_____

_____

_____

_____

4. Do you deserve to live?

Why? Why not? Did they ever tell you, "You deserve to die"? If so, was this part of your religious upbringing?

_____

_____

_____

_____

5. What do you have to live for?

What is the purpose in your life? What meaning have you created?

_____

_____

_____

_____

6. What do you deserve?

"I deserve love and joy and all good." Or do you feel deep down that you deserve nothing? Why? Where did the message come from? Are you willing to let it go? What are you willing to put in its place? Remember, these are thoughts, and thoughts can be changed.

_____

_____

_____

_____

You can see that personal power is affected by the way we perceive our deservability. Try this treatment. Put most simply, treatments are positive statements made in any given situation to establish new thought patterns, and dissolve old ones.

DESERVABILITY TREATMENT

I am deserving. I deserve all good. Not some, not a little bit, but all good. I now move past all negative, restricting thoughts. I release and let go of the limitations of my parents. I love them, and I go beyond them. I am not their negative opinions, nor their limiting beliefs. I am not bound by any of the fears or prejudices of the current society I live in. I no longer identify with limitation of any kind.

In my mind, I have total freedom. I now move into a new space of consciousness, where I am willing to see myself differently. I am willing to create new thoughts about myself and about my life. My new thinking becomes new experiences.

I now know and affirm that I am at one with the Prospering Power of the Universe. As such, I now prosper in a number of ways. The totality of possibilities lies before me. I deserve life, a good life. I deserve love, an abundance of love. I deserve good health. I deserve to live comfortably and to prosper. I deserve joy and happiness. I deserve freedom to be all that I can be. I deserve more than that. I deserve all good.

The Universe is more than willing to manifest my new beliefs. And I accept this abundant life with joy, pleasure, and gratitude. For I am deserving. I accept it; I know it to be true.

2

WHO ARE YOU?
WHAT DO YOU BELIEVE?

"I see myself with eyes of love and I am safe."

In this section I would like us to look at ourselves and at our beliefs. We all have many positive things we believe, and we want to continue to reinforce these. And many of our beliefs are negative and continue to contribute to uncomfortable experiences. It is impossible for us to change any limiting beliefs unless we know what they are. Look at this list of words. Write down what they mean to you. For example, do you believe that:

MEN...

> *Men are strong.*
> *Men are bossy.*
> *Men are smart.*

WOMEN...

> *Women get paid less.*
> *Women have to clean the house.*
> *Women are soft and tender.*

LOVE...

> *Love is for the birds.*
> *I love to be loved.*
> *Love equals loss and heartbreak.*

SEX...

> *Sex is fun.*
> *Sex is only for marriage.*
> *Sex is painful.*

WORK...

> *Work is boring.*
> *Bosses are mean.*
> *Other people have good jobs.*

MONEY...

> *There is never enough.*
> *I'm afraid of money.*
> *Money is for spending.*

SUCCESS...

> *Success is out of my reach.*
> *Only the rich are successful.*
> *I can succeed in little things.*

FAILURE...

> *When I make a mistake, I am a failure.*
> *Failure means doing it wrong.*
> *Failure is something to learn from.*

GOD...

> *God loves me.*
> *I am one with God.*
> *I'm afraid of God.*

Now it's your turn. Think of all the things these words mean to you. Make the list as long as you like.

MEN...

_____

_____

_____

_____

_____

_____

WOMEN...

_____

_____

_____

_____

_____

_____

LOVE...

_____

_____

_____

_____

_____

_____

SEX...

_____

_____

_____

_____

_____

_____

_____

WORK...

_____

_____

_____

_____

_____

_____

_____

MONEY...

_____

_____

_____

_____

_____

_____

_____

SUCCESS...

_____

_____

_____

_____

_____

_____

_____

FAILURE...

_____

_____

_____

_____

_____

_____

_____

GOD...

_____

_____

_____

_____

_____

_____

_____

Now, notice the areas that are difficult for you. Do you have conflicting beliefs? How many of your answers are negative? Put a star beside these answers. Do you really want to continue to build your life on these convictions? Be aware that someone taught you these ideas. Now that you have seen them, you can choose to let them go.

EXERCISE: *Your Story*

This might be the time for you to write a brief story of your life. Begin with your childhood. Use more paper if you need to.

_____

_____

_____

_____

_____

_____

_____

_____

_____

_____

_____

_____

_____

_____

_____

_____

_____

What other negative beliefs could you have rattling around in your subconscious mind? Allow them to come up. You may be surprised at what you find. How many negative messages did you notice when you wrote your story? Each negative belief that surfaces is a treasure. "Ah ha! I have found you. You are the one that has been causing me all this trouble. Now I can eliminate you."

Other negative beliefs:

_____

_____

_____

_____

This would be a good time to pick up your hand mirror and to look in your eyes and affirm your "willingness" to release all these old negative messages and beliefs. Breathe deeply as you do this and speak aloud if you can. "I am willing to release all old negative concepts and beliefs that are no longer nourishing me." Repeat it several times.

Inner Child

Many of us have an inner child who is lost and lonely and feels so rejected. Perhaps the only contact we have had with our inner child for a long times is to scold it and criticize it. Then we wonder why we are unhappy. We cannot reject a part of us and still be in harmony within. Part of healing is to gather all the parts of ourselves so we may be whole and complete. Let's do some work to connect with these neglected inner parts of ourselves.

Find a Photo

Find a photo of yourself as a child. If you don't have one, ask your parents to send you one. Study this picture closely. What do you see? It may be joy, pain, sorrow, anger, or fear. Do you love this child? Can you relate to it? I took a small photo of myself at the age of five and had it blown up to 12 by 15 so that I could really see my little girl.

Write a few words about your inner child.

_____

_____

_____

_____

_____

_____

_____

Draw a Picture

Take several crayons, felt-tipped pens, or colored pencils. You can use the paper in this workbook or get a larger piece of your own. Use your nondominant hand (the one you don't write with), and draw a picture of yourself as a child.

What does this picture tell you? What colors did you use? What is the child doing? Describe this picture.

_____

_____

_____

_____

Talk to Your Inner Child

Take a little time now to talk to your inner child. Discover more about this child. Ask questions.

1. What do you like?

_____

_____

_____

_____

2. What do you dislike?

_____

_____

_____

_____

3. What frightens you?

_____

_____

_____

_____

4. How do you feel?

_____

_____

_____

_____

5. What do you need?

_____

_____

_____

_____

6. How can I help you feel safe?

_____

_____

_____

_____

7. How can I make you happy?

_____

_____

_____

_____

Have a good conversation with your inner child. Be there for that child. Embrace it and love it, and do what you can to take care of its needs. Be sure to let it know that no matter what happens, you will always be there. You can begin to create a happy childhood. This exercise works best with your eyes closed.

POWER POINTS

"I believe in my own power to change."

This small section may be the most important part of this book. Continually refer to it as you explore the various areas of your life. Make several lists of these seven points. Place these lists where you can see them. Read them often. Memorize them. When these concepts become part of your belief system, you will have a different perspective on life.

1. We are each responsible for our experiences.

2. Every thought we think is creating our future.

3. Everyone is dealing with the damaging patterns of resentment, criticism, guilt, and self-hatred.

4. These are only thoughts and thoughts can be changed.

5. We need to release the past and forgive everyone.

6. Self-approval and self-acceptance in the "now" are the keys to positive changes.

7. The point of power is always in the present moment.

As you do the exercises in this workbook, keep coming back to these seven points. Do not just get stuck in your specific problems. When you really accept these ideas and make them a part of your belief system, you become "powerful," and the problems will often solve themselves. The object is to change what you believe about yourself and the world you live in.

It is not the people, places, and things that are creating a problem for you; it is how you are "perceiving and reacting" to these life experiences. Take responsibility for your own life. Do not give your power away. Learn to understand more of your inner, spiritual-self, and operate under that power that created only good for you.

"I give myself permission to learn."

PART II

THE PROCESS

3

HEALTH

"I restore and maintain my body at optimum health."

Health Checklist

- ☐ I get three colds every year.
- ☐ My energy level is low.
- ☐ I heal slowly.
- ☐ My allergies act up constantly.
- ☐ Heart dis-ease runs in my family.
- ☐ I get one illness after another.
- ☐ My back gives me constant pain.
- ☐ These headaches never go away.
- ☐ I'm always constipated.
- ☐ I have sore feet.
- ☐ I'm always hurting my body.

*H*ow many of these sound like you? Let's look at our beliefs about health.

I believe that we contribute to every "illness" in our body. The body, as with everything else in life, is a mirror of our inner thoughts and beliefs. Our body is always talking to us, if we will only take the time to listen. Every cell within our bodies responds to every single thought we think.

When we discover what the mental pattern is behind an illness, we have a chance to change the pattern and, therefore, the dis-ease. Most people do not want to be sick on a conscious level, yet every dis-ease that we have is a teacher. Illness is the body's way of telling us that there is a false idea in our consciousness. Something that we are believing, saying, doing, or thinking is not for our highest good. I always picture the body tugging at us saying, "Please—pay attention!"

Sometimes people *do* want to be sick. In our society, we've made illness a legitimate way to avoid responsibility or unpleasant situations. If we can't learn to say "no," then we may have to invent a dis-ease to say "no" for us.

I read an interesting report a few years back. It stated that only 30 percent of patients follow their doctor's instructions. According to Dr. John Harrison, author of the fascinating book *Love Your Disease*, many people go to doctors only to have their acute symptoms relieved, so that they can tolerate their dis-ease. It is as if an unwritten, subconscious agreement exists between doctor and patient: the doctor agrees not to cure the patient if the patient pretends to do something about his or her condition. Also in this agreement, one person gets to pay, and the other becomes the authority figure, and so, both parties are satisfied.

True healing involves body, mind, and spirit. I believe that if we "cure" an illness, yet do not address the emotional and spiritual issues that surround that illness, it will only manifest itself again.

EXERCISE: *Releasing Your Health Problems*

Are you willing to release the need that has contributed to your health problems? Once again, when we have a condition that we want to change, the first thing that we have to do is to say so. Say: "I am willing to release the need in me that has created this condition." Say it again. Say it looking in the mirror. Say it every time that you think about your condition. It is the first step in creating a change.

1. List all of your mother's illnesses.

_____

_____

_____

_____

2. List all of your father's illnesses.

_____

_____

_____

_____

3. List all of your illnesses.

_____

_____

_____

_____

4. Do you see a connection?

_____

_____

_____

_____

EXERCISE: *Health and Dis-ease*

Let's examine some of your beliefs about health and dis-ease. Answer the following questions. Be as open and honest as you can.

1. What do you remember about your childhood illnesses?

_____

_____

_____

_____

2. What did you learn from your parents about illness?

_____

_____

_____

_____

3. What, if anything, did you enjoy about being sick as a child?

_____

_____

_____

_____

4. Is there a belief about illness from your childhood that you are still acting on today?

_____

_____

_____

_____

5. How have you contributed to the state of your health?

_____

_____

_____

_____

6. Would you like your condition to change? If so, in what way?

_____

_____

_____

_____

EXERCISE: *Your Beliefs About Sickness*

Complete the following statements as honestly as you can.

1. The way I make myself sick is...

_____

_____

_____

_____

2. I get sick when I try to avoid...

_____

_____

_____

_____

3. When I get sick, I always want to...

_____

_____

_____

_____

4. When I was sick as a child, my mother always...

_____

_____

_____

_____

5. My greatest fear when I am sick is...

_____

_____

_____

_____

EXERCISE: *The Power of Affirmations*

Let's discover the power of written affirmations! Writing an affirmation can intensify its power. In the space below, write a positive affirmation about your health 25 times. You may create your own, or use one of the following:

1. My healing is already in process.

2. I listen with love to my body's messages.

3. My health is radiant, vibrant and dynamic now.

4. I am grateful for my perfect health.

5. I deserve good health.

1. _____

2. _____

3. _____

4. _____

5. _____

6. _____

7. _____

8. _____

9. _____

10. _____

11. _____

12. _____

13. _____

14. _____

15. _____

16. _____

17. _____

18. _____

19. _____

20. _____

21. _____

22. _____

23. _____

24. _____

25. _____

EXERCISE: *Self-Worth*

Let's examine the issue of self-worth. Answer the following questions, and after each one, create a positive affirmation.

1. **Do I deserve good health?**

   Example:
   No. Illness runs in my family.

YOUR EXAMPLE:

_____

_____

_____

_____

_____

Sample Affirmation:
I accept and deserve perfect health now.

YOUR AFFIRMATION:

_____

_____

_____

_____

_____

2. What do I fear most about my health?

Example:
I am afraid that I will get sick.

YOUR EXAMPLE:

_____

_____

_____

_____

_____

Sample Affirmation:
It is safe to be well now. I am always loved.

YOUR AFFIRMATION:

_____

_____

_____

_____

_____

3. **What am I "getting" from this belief?**

Example:
I don't have to be responsible.

YOUR EXAMPLE:

_____

_____

_____

_____

Sample Affirmation:
I am confident and secure. Life is easy for me.

YOUR AFFIRMATION:

_____

_____

_____

_____

_____

4. What do I fear would happen if I let go of this belief?

Example:
I would have to grow up.

YOUR EXAMPLE:

_____

_____

_____

_____

_____

_____

Sample Affirmation:
It is safe to be an adult.

YOUR AFFIRMATION:

_____

_____

_____

_____

_____

_____

Review the belief checklist taken from page 27, then study the affirmations corresponding to each belief. Make these affirmations part of your daily routine. Say them often in the car, at work, in the mirror, or any time you feel your negative beliefs surfacing.

If You Believe:	*Your Affirmation Is:*
I get three colds every year.	*I am safe and secure at all times. Love surrounds me and protects me.*
My energy level is low.	*I am filled with energy and enthusiasm.*
I heal slowly.	*My body heals rapidly.*
My allergies act up constantly.	*The world is safe. I am safe. I am at peace with life.*
Heart dis-ease runs in my family.	*I am healthy and whole.*
I get one illness after another.	*Good health is mine now. I release the past.*
My back gives me constant pain.	*Life loves and supports me. I am safe.*
These headaches never go away.	*My mind is at peace and all is well.*
I'm always constipated.	*I allow life to flow through me.*
I have sore feet.	*I am willing to move forward with ease.*
I'm always hurting my body.	*I am gentle with my body. I love myself.*

"I give myself permission to be well."

POWER POINTS

1. We are each responsible for our experiences.

2. Every thought we think is creating our future.

3. Everyone is dealing with the damaging patterns of resentment, criticism, guilt, and self-hatred.

4. These are only thoughts and thoughts can be changed.

5. We need to release the past and forgive everyone, including ourselves.

6. Self-approval and self-acceptance in the "now" are the keys to positive changes.

7. The point of power is always in the present moment.

4

FEELING GOOD

"It is my divine right to be comfortable."

Feeling Good Checklist

- ☐ I'm anxious all of the time.
- ☐ I'm frightened of people.
- ☐ My loneliness is intense.
- ☐ I have difficulty expressing my feelings.
- ☐ My temper is out of control.
- ☐ I can't focus on anything.
- ☐ Everyone is against me.
- ☐ I can't assert myself.
- ☐ I feel like a failure.
- ☐ I want to hide under the covers.

Can you identify with any of these feelings? You may need to work on your emotional well-being.

Emotional problems are among the most painful of all. Occasionally we may feel angry, sad, lonely, guilty, anxious, or frightened. When these feelings take over and become predominant, our life can become an emotional battleground.

What we *do* with our feelings is important. Are we going to act them out? Will we punish others or force our will upon them? Will we abuse ourselves in some way?

The belief that we are *not good enough* is often at the root of these problems. Good mental health begins with *loving the self*. When we love and approve of ourselves *completely*, the good and the so-called bad, we can begin to change.

Part of self-acceptance is releasing other people's opinions. Many of the things we have chosen to believe about ourselves have absolutely no basis in truth.

For example, a young man named Eric was a client of mine several years ago when I was seeing people privately. He was devastatingly handsome and made a good living as a model. He told me what a hard time he had going to the gym because he felt ugly.

As we worked together, we discovered that a neighborhood bully from his childhood used to call him "ugly." This person would also beat him up and constantly threaten him. In order to be left alone and to feel safe, Eric began to hide. He bought into the fact that he was not good enough. In his mind, he was ugly.

Through mirror work, self-love, and positive affirmations, Eric has improved tremendously. His feelings of anxiety may come and go, but he now has some tools to work with.

Remember, feelings of inadequacy start with negative thoughts that we have about ourselves. However, these thoughts have no power over us unless *we* act upon them. Thoughts are only words strung together. They have *no meaning whatsoever*. Only WE give meaning to them. We give meaning to them by focusing on the negative messages over and over again in our minds. We believe the worst about ourselves. And *we* choose what *kind* of meaning we give to them.

Whatever pain we might be in, let's choose thoughts that nourish and support us.

MIRROR WORK

Do you believe that you deserve peace and serenity in your emotional life? If you don't, you won't allow yourself to have it. Look into your mirror again and say, "I deserve inner peace, and I accept it now." Say it a few times.

1. What kind of feelings come up for you?

_____

_____

_____

_____

2. How does your body feel?

_____

_____

_____

_____

3. Does it feel true, or do you still feel unworthy?

_____

_____

_____

_____

If you have any negative feelings in your body, then affirm: "I release the pattern in my consciousness that is creating resistance to my good. I deserve to feel good."

Repeat this until you feel acceptance. Do this several days in a row. You may feel funny doing some of these exercises. You may wonder how they might possibly change you. I have seen them work for many people. Taking one step at a time will accomplish wonders.

EXERCISE: *Have Fun With Your Inner Child*

When you are in a state of anxiety or fear that keeps you from functioning, you may have abandoned your inner child. Think of some ways in which you can reconnect with your inner child. What could you do for fun? What could you do that is JUST FOR YOU?

List 15 ways in which you could have fun with your inner child. You may enjoy reading good books, going to the movies, gardening, keeping a journal, or taking a hot bath. How about some "child-like" activities? Really take the time to think. You could run on the beach, go to a playground and swing on a swing, you could draw pictures with crayons, or climb a tree. Once you have made your list, try doing at least one activity each day. Let the healing begin!

1. _____

2. _____

3. _____

4. _____

5. _____

6. _____

7. _____

8. _____

9. _____

10. _____

11. _____

12. _____

13. _____

14. _____

15. _____

Look at all you have discovered! Keep going—you can create such fun for you and your child! Feel the relationship between the two of you healing.

EXERCISE: *Your Thankful List*

What are you grateful for? How do you begin your day? What is the first thing that you say in the morning? Is it positive or negative? I spend about 10 minutes being thankful for all of the good in my life. List at least 10 things in your life that you are grateful for. You may take a month to write this list. Don't worry—there is no time limit. You may always add to the list. Close your eyes and really think before you write.

1. _____

2. _____

3. _____

4. _____

5. _____

6. _____

7. _____

8. _____

9. _____

10. _____

EXERCISE: *Positive Feelings*

Let's examine your feelings. In the space below, write 50 positive things about yourself. Pay attention to your feelings while you are doing the exercise. Is there resistance? Is it hard for you to see yourself in a positive light? Continue on! Remember how powerful you are!

1. _____

2. _____

3. _____

4. _____

5. _____

6. _____

7. _____

8. _____

9. _____

10. _____

11. _____

12. _____

13. _____

14. _____

15. _____

16. _____

17. _____

18. _____

19. _____

20. _____

21. _____

22. _____

23. _____

24. _____

25. _____

26. _____

27. _____

28. _____

29. _____

30. _____

31. _____

32. _____

33. _____

34. _____

35. _____

36. _____

37. _____

38. _____

39. _____

40. _____

41. _____

42. _____

43. _____

44. _____

45. _____

46. _____

47. _____

48. _____

49. _____

50. _____

Refer to the checklist on the next page taken from page 39. Find the affirmation corresponding to each belief. Make these affirmations part of your daily schedule.

If You Believe:	*Your Affirmation Is:*
I am anxious all of the time.	*I am at peace.*
I'm frightened of people.	*Loving others is easy when I love and accept myself.*
My loneliness is intense.	*I am safe, it's only change.*
I have difficulty expressing myself.	*It is safe to express my feelings.*
My temper is out of control.	*I am at peace with myself and life.*
I can't focus on anything.	*My inner vision is clear and unclouded.*
Everyone is against me.	*I am loveable and everybody loves me.*
I can't assert myself.	*I love who I am and I assert my power wisely.*
I feel like a failure.	*My life is a success.*
I want to hide under the covers.	*I now go beyond my old fears and limitations.*

"I give myself permission to relax."

POWER POINTS

1. We are each responsible for our experiences.

2. Every thought we think is creating our future.

3. Everyone is dealing with the damaging patterns of resentment, criticism, guilt, and self-hatred.

4. These are only thoughts and thoughts can be changed.

5. We need to release the past and forgive everyone, including ourselves.

6. Self-approval and self-acceptance in the "now" are the keys to positive changes.

7. The point of power is always in the present moment.

FEARS AND PHOBIAS

"Fears are merely thoughts and thoughts can be released."

Fears and Phobias Checklist

- ☐ I am afraid to leave the house.
- ☐ It wouldn't work for me.
- ☐ Growing older frightens me.
- ☐ I am afraid of flying.
- ☐ People scare me.
- ☐ What if I become homeless?
- ☐ Driving a car makes me claustrophobic.
- ☐ What if I have a painful death?
- ☐ I'm afraid of being alone.
- ☐ I'll never be able to face old age.

*H*ow many of these sound like you? Let's examine our mechanisms behind fear.

In any given situation, I believe that we have a choice between love and fear. We experience fear of change, fear of not changing, fear of the future, and fear of taking a chance. We fear intimacy, and we fear being alone. We fear letting people know what we need and who we are, and we fear letting go of the past.

At the other end of the spectrum we have love. Love is the miracle we are all looking for. Loving ourselves works miracles in our lives. I am not talking about vanity or arrogance, for that is not love. That is fear. I am talking about having a great respect for ourselves and a gratitude for the miracle of our body and our mind.

Remind yourself when you are frightened that you are not loving and trusting yourself. Not feeling "good enough" interferes with the decision-making process. How can you make a good decision when you are not sure about yourself?

Susan Jeffers, in her marvelous book, *Feel the Fear and Do It Anyway*, states that "if everybody feels fear when approaching something totally new in life, yet so many are out there 'doing it' despite the fear, then we must conclude that *fear is not the problem.*" She goes on to say that the real issue is not the fear, but how we *hold* the fear. We can approach it from a position of power or helplessness. The fact that we have the fear becomes irrelevant.

We see what we *think* the problem is, and then we find out what the *real* problem is. Not feeling "good enough" and a lack of self-love is the real problem.

We are always perfect, always beautiful, and ever-changing. We are doing the best we can with the understanding, knowledge, and awareness that we have. As we grow and change more and more, our "best" will only get better and better.

EXERCISE: *Letting Go*

As you read this exercise, take a deep breath and, as you exhale, allow the tension to leave your body. Let your scalp and your forehead and your face relax. Your head need not be tense in order for you to read. Let your tongue and your throat and your shoulders relax. You can hold a book with relaxed arms and hands. Do that now. Let your back and your abdomen and your pelvis relax. Let your breathing be at peace as you relax your legs and feet.

Do you feel a noticeable change in your body since you started reading the previous paragraph? Notice how much you hold on. If you are holding on with your body, you are holding on with your mind.

In this relaxed, comfortable position, say to yourself, "I am willing to let go. I release. I let go. I release all tension. I release all fear. I release all anger. I release all guilt. I release all sadness. I let go of old limitations. I let go and I am at peace. I am at peace with myself. I am at peace with the process of life. I am safe."

Go over this exercise two or three times. Feel the ease of letting go. Repeat it whenever thoughts of difficulty come up. It takes a little practice for the routine to become a part of you. Once you are familiar with this exercise, you can do it anywhere at any time. You will be able to relax completely in any situation.

EXERCISE: *Fears and Affirmations*

After each category listed below, write down your greatest fear. Then, think of a positive affirmation that would correspond to it.

1. Career

Example:
I am afraid that no one will ever see my value.

YOUR FEAR:

_____

_____

_____

_____

Sample Affirmation:
Everybody at work appreciates me.

YOUR AFFIRMATION:

_____

_____

_____

_____

2. Living Situation

Example:
I'll never have a place of my own.

YOUR FEAR:

_____

_____

_____

_____

Sample Affirmation:
There is a perfect home for me and I accept it now.

YOUR AFFIRMATION:

_____

_____

_____

_____

3. Family Relations

Example:
My parents won't accept me the way I am.

YOUR FEAR:

_____

_____

_____

_____

Sample Affirmation:
I accept my parents and they in turn accept and love me.

YOUR AFFIRMATION:

_____

_____

_____

_____

4. Money

Example:
I am afraid of being poor.

YOUR FEAR:

_____

_____

_____

_____

Sample Affirmation:
I trust that all my needs will be taken care of.

YOUR AFFIRMATION:

_____

_____

_____

_____

5. Physical appearance

Example:
I think that I'm fat and unattractive.

YOUR FEAR:

_____

_____

_____

Sample Affirmation:
I release the need to criticize my body.

YOUR AFFIRMATION:

_____

_____

_____

6. Sex

Example:
I am afraid that I will have to "perform."

YOUR FEAR:

_____

_____

_____

_____

Sample Affirmation:
I am relaxed and I flow with life easily and effortlessly.

YOUR AFFIRMATION:

_____

_____

_____

_____

7. Health

Example:
I am afraid of being sick and unable to take care of myself.

YOUR FEAR:

_____

_____

_____

_____

Sample Affirmation:
I will always attract all the help I need.

YOUR AFFIRMATION:

_____

_____

_____

_____

8. Relationships

Example:
I don't think that anyone will ever love me.

YOUR FEAR:

_____

_____

_____

_____

Sample Affirmation:
Love and acceptance are mine. I love myself.

YOUR AFFIRMATION:

_____

_____

_____

_____

9. Old Age

Example:
I am afraid of getting old.

YOUR FEAR:

_____

_____

_____

_____

Sample Affirmation:
Every age has its infinite possibilities.

YOUR AFFIRMATION:

_____

_____

_____

_____

10. Death and Dying

Example:
What if there is no life after death?

YOUR FEAR:

_____

_____

_____

_____

Sample Affirmation:
I trust the process of life. I am on an endless journey through eternity.

YOUR AFFIRMATION:

_____

_____

_____

_____

EXERCISE: *Positive Affirmations*

Choose an area of fear from the last exercise that is most immediate for you. Using visualization, see yourself going through the fear, with a positive outcome. See yourself feeling free and at peace. Write down a positive affirmation 25 times. Remember the power you are tapping into!

1. _____

2. _____

3. _____

4. _____

5. _____

6. _____

7. _____

8. _____

9. _____

10. _____

11. _____

12. _____

13. _____

14. _____

15. _____

16. _____

17. _____

18. _____

19. _____

20. _____

21. _____

22. _____

23. _____

24. _____

25. _____

Review the belief checklist below taken from page 49, then study the affirmations corresponding to each belief. Make these affirmations part of your daily routine. Say them often in the car, at work, in the mirror, or any time you feel your negative beliefs surfacing.

If You Believe:	*Your Affirmation Is:*
I am afraid to leave the house.	*I am always safe and protected.*
It wouldn't work for me.	*My decisions are always perfect for me.*
Growing older frightens me.	*My age is perfect and I enjoy each new moment.*
I am afraid of flying.	*I center myself in safety and accept the perfection of my life.*
People scare me.	*I am loved and safe wherever I go.*
What if I become homeless?	*I am at home in the universe.*
Driving a car makes me claustrophobic.	*I relax and move with joy, ease, and comfort.*
What if I have a painful death?	*I will die peacefully and comfortably at the right time.*
I'm afraid of being alone.	*I express love and I will always attract love wherever I go.*

"I give myself permission to be at peace."

POWER POINTS

1. We are each responsible for our experiences.

2. Every thought we think is creating our future.

3. Everyone is dealing with the damaging patterns of resentment, criticism, guilt, and self-hatred.

4. These are only thoughts and thoughts can be changed.

5. We need to release the past and forgive everyone, including ourselves.

6. Self-approval and self-acceptance in the "now" are the keys to positive changes.

7. The point of power is always in the present moment.

6

ANGER

"I accept all my emotions with love."

Anger Checklist

- ☐ I am afraid of anger.
- ☐ If I get angry, I will lose control.
- ☐ I have no right to be angry.
- ☐ Anger is bad.
- ☐ When someone is angry, I get scared.
- ☐ It's not safe to be angry.
- ☐ My parents won't allow me to express anger.
- ☐ I won't be loved if I get angry.
- ☐ I have to hide my anger.
- ☐ Stuffing anger makes me sick.
- ☐ I have never been angry.
- ☐ If I get angry, I will hurt someone.

Do you recognize any of these feelings? Anger may be one of your big barriers.

Anger is a natural and normal emotion. Babies get furious, express their fury and then it's over. Many of us have learned that it's not nice, or polite, or acceptable for us to be angry. We learn to swallow our angry feelings. They settle in our bodies, in the joints and muscles. They accumulate and become resentment. Layer upon layer of buried anger turned into resentment can contribute to dis-eases like arthritis, assorted pains, and even cancer.

We need to acknowledge all our feelings, including anger, and find positive ways to express these feelings. We don't have to hit people or dump on them, yet we can say simply and clearly, "This makes me angry." Or "I am angry at what you did." If it is not appropriate to say this, we still have many options: we can scream into a pillow. Beat the bed. Kick pillows. Run. Yell in the car with the windows rolled up. Play tennis. These are all healthy outlets.

1. What was the pattern of anger in your family?

_____

_____

_____

_____

2. What did your father do with his anger?

_____

_____

_____

_____

3. What did your mother do with her anger?

_____

_____

_____

_____

_____

_____

4. What did your brothers or sisters do with their anger?

_____

_____

_____

_____

5. Was there a family scapegoat?

_____

_____

_____

_____

6. What did you do with your anger as a child?

_____

_____

_____

_____

7. Did you express your anger or did you stuff it?

_____

_____

_____

_____

_____

_____

_____

8. What method did you use to hold it in?

_____

_____

_____

_____

9. Were you:
   an overeater? ....☐ Yes   ☐ No
   always sick? ....☐ Yes   ☐ No
   accident prone? ....☐ Yes   ☐ No
   getting into fights? ....☐ Yes   ☐ No
   a poor student? ....☐ Yes   ☐ No
   crying all of the time? ....☐ Yes   ☐ No

10. How do you handle your anger now?

_____

_____

_____

_____

11. Do you see a family pattern?

_____

_____

_____

_____

_____

_____

12. Which family member are you like when it comes to expressing anger?

_____

_____

_____

_____

13. Do you have a "right" to be angry?

_____

_____

_____

_____

14. Why not? Who said so?

_____

_____

_____

_____

15. Can you give yourself permission to express all your feelings in appropriate ways?

_____

_____

_____

_____

A quick and simple thing to do when you are overwhelmed with your feelings is to jump up and down several times saying in a loud voice, "Yes! No! Get off my back! Yes! No! Get off my back!" Try it. It works wonders for a quick release.

If you have a lot of buried anger, you may be a person who walks around being angry all the time. The anger is smoldering just under the surface. The smallest thing will set it off. You may not express this anger, but you will mutter under your breath and have lots of resentful, judgmental thoughts. You may be a person who criticizes everyone around you. And if you do, you certainly will criticize yourself, too. So you may ask yourself:

1. What do I get from being angry all the time?

_____

_____

_____

_____

_____

2. What happens if I let go of my anger?

_____

_____

_____

_____

_____

3. Am I willing to forgive and be free?

_____

_____

_____

_____

_____

_____

_____

EXERCISE: *Write a Letter*

Think of someone who you are still angry with. Perhaps it is an old anger. Write this person a letter. Tell them all your grievances and how you feel. Don't hold back. Really express yourself. Use additional paper if you need it.

_____

_____

_____

_____

_____

_____

_____

_____

_____

When you have finished the letter, read it once. Then fold it and on the outside write: "What I really want is your love and approval." Then burn the letter and release it.

MIRROR WORK

Take another person, or the same person, you are angry with. Sit down in front of a mirror. Be sure to have some tissues nearby. Look into your own eyes and see the other person. Tell them what you are so angry about.

When you are finished, tell them, "What I really want is your love and approval." We are all seeking love and approval. That's what we want from everyone, and that's what everyone wants from us. Love and approval brings harmony into our lives.

In order to be free, we need to release the old ties that bind us. So once again look into the mirror and affirm to yourself, "I am willing to release the need to be an angry person." Notice if you are really willing to let go or do you still want to hang on to the past.

Review the beliefs checklist below, taken from page 61. Next to them are the corresponding affirmations. Practice them in the car, while brushing your teeth in the morning, in the mirror, or anytime you feel your negatives coming to the surface.

If You Believe:	*Your Affirmation Is:*
I am afraid of anger.	*I acknowledge all my feelings. It is safe for me to recognize my anger.*
If I get angry, I will lose control.	*I express my anger in appropriate places and ways.*
I have no right to be angry.	*All my emotions are acceptable.*
Anger is bad.	*Anger is normal and natural.*
When someone is angry I get scared.	*I comfort my inner child and we are safe.*
It's not safe to be angry.	*I am safe with all my emotions.*
My parents won't allow me to express anger.	*I move beyond my parents' limitations.*
I won't be loved if I get angry.	*The more honest I am, the more I am loved.*
I have to hide my anger.	*I express my anger in appropriate ways.*
Stuffing anger makes me sick.	*I allow myself freedom with all my emotions, including anger.*
I have never been angry.	*Healthy expressions of anger keep me healthy.*
If I get angry I will hurt someone.	*Everyone is safe with me when I express my emotions.*

"I give myself permission to acknowledge my feelings."

POWER POINTS

1. We are each responsible for our experiences.

2. Every thought we think is creating our future.

3. Everyone is dealing with the damaging patterns of resentment, criticism, guilt, and self-hatred.

4. These are only thoughts and thoughts can be changed.

5. We need to release the past and forgive everyone, including ourselves.

6. Self-approval and self-acceptance in the "now" are the keys to positive changes.

7. The point of power is always in the present moment.

CRITICISM AND JUDGMENT

Criticism and Judgment Checklist

- ☐ Why are there so many bad drivers?
- ☐ People are so stupid.
- ☐ I'm such a jerk.
- ☐ I'd do it if I weren't so fat.
- ☐ Those are the ugliest clothes I've ever seen.
- ☐ They'll never be able to finish the job.
- ☐ I'm such a klutz.
- ☐ The people around here are such slobs.
- ☐ My neighbors are so noisy.
- ☐ Nobody asks me what I think.
- ☐ Can you believe that old car that she drives?
- ☐ I hate his laugh.

Does your inner dialogue sound like this? Is your inner voice constantly picking, picking, picking? Are you seeing the world through critical eyes? Do you judge everything? Do you stand in self-righteousness?

Most of us have such a strong habit of judgment and criticism that we cannot easily break it. It is also the most important issue to work on immediately. We will never be able to really love ourselves until we go beyond the need to make life wrong.

As a little baby you were so open to life. You looked at the world with eyes of wonder. Unless something was scary or someone harmed you, you accepted life just as it was. Later, as you grew up, you began to accept the opinions of others and to make them your own. You learned how to criticize.

1. What was your family pattern?

_____

_____

_____

_____

_____

2. What did you learn about criticism from your mother?

_____

_____

_____

_____

_____

3. What were the things she criticized?

_____

_____

_____

_____

_____

4. Did she criticize you?

_____

_____

_____

_____

5. What for?

_____

_____

_____

_____

6. When was your father judgmental?

_____

_____

_____

_____

7. Did he judge himself?

_____

_____

_____

_____

_____

_____

_____

8. How did your father judge you?

_____

_____

_____

_____

9. Was it a family pattern to criticize each other?

_____

_____

_____

_____

10. How and when did they do this?

_____

_____

_____

_____

11. When was the first time you remember being criticized?

_____

_____

_____

_____

_____

_____

12. How did your family judge the neighbors?

_____

_____

_____

_____

_____

13. Did you have loving, supportive teachers at school? Or were they always telling you what was lacking in you? What sort of things *did* they tell you?

_____

_____

_____

_____

_____

14. Can you begin to see where you might have picked up this pattern? Who was the most critical person in your childhood?

_____

_____

_____

_____

_____

Perhaps you were led to believe that you need to criticize yourself in order to grow and change. I do not agree with that concept at all!

I believe that criticism shrivels our spirits. It only enforces the belief that "we are not good enough." It certainly does not bring out the best in us.

EXERCISE: *Replacing Your "Shoulds"*

As I have said many times, I believe that "should" is one of the most damaging words in our language. Every time we use it, we are, in effect, saying "wrong." Either we are wrong, or we were wrong, or we are going to be wrong. I would like to take the word "should" out of our vocabulary forever, and replace it with the word "could." "Could" gives us choice and we are never wrong. Think of five things that you "should" do.

I SHOULD:

1. _____

2. _____

3. _____

4. _____

5. _____

Replace SHOULD with COULD.

I COULD:

1. _____

2. _____

3. _____

4. _____

5. _____

Now, ask yourself, "Why haven't I?" You may find that you have been berating yourself for years for something that you never wanted to do in the first place, or for something that was never your idea. How many "shoulds" can you drop from your list?

EXERCISE: *Your Critical List*

Make a list of five things you criticize yourself for:

1. _____

2. _____

3. _____

4. _____

5. _____

Now, go back over that list and put a date beside each one—the date that you began to add that item to your "get wrong" list.

Isn't it amazing how long you have been picking on yourself for the same thing? This habit has not produced any positive changes has it? Exactly. Criticism doesn't work! It only makes you feel bad. So, be willing to stop it.

In order for a child to grow and blossom, it needs love, acceptance, and praise. We can be shown "better" ways to do things without making the way we do it "wrong." The child inside of you still needs that love and approval.

"I love you and know that you are doing the best you can."

"You are perfect just as you are."

"You become more wonderful every day."

"I approve of you."

"Let's see if we can find a better way to do this."

"Growing and changing is fun, and we can do it together."

These are words that children want to hear. It makes them feel good. When they feel good, they do their best. They unfold beautifully.

If your child, or your inner child, is used to constantly being "wrong," it may take awhile for them to accept the new, positive words. If you make a definite decision to release criticism, and are consistent, you can work miracles.

Give yourself one month of talking to your inner child in positive ways. Use the affirmations listed above. Make up a list of some of your own. Carry a list of these affirmations with you. When you notice yourself becoming judgmental, take out the list and read it two or three times. Better yet, do it aloud in front of a mirror.

EXERCISE:　*Who Annoys You?*

Who else do you belittle? List five of their names and what you find most annoying about them.

Example:
George. He never smiles.
Sally. Her makeup is just terrible.

1. _____

2. _____

3. _____

4. _____

5. _____

Now, take those same people and make another list. This time, find something positive to say about each person—something that you can praise. Look for it. Even a small thing will do.

1. _____

2. _____

3. _____

4. _____

5. _____

From now on, every time you think of these people, use a sentence on your list to praise them. Keep your mind filled with positive thoughts. Make a habit of allowing only positive comments come out of your mouth. If you want to change your life, you need to control your mouth.

EXERCISE:　*Listen to Yourself*

This exercise requires a tape recorder. Tape your telephone conversations for a week or so—just your voice. When the tape is filled on both sides, sit down and listen to it. Listen to not only what you say, but the way you say it. What are your beliefs? Who and what do you criticize? Which parent, if any, do you sound like?

As you release the need to pick on yourself all the time, you will notice that you no longer criticize others so much.

When you make it okay to be yourself, then you automatically allow others to be themselves. Their little habits no longer bother you so much. You release the need to "change them" as you want to be. As you stop judging others, they release the need to judge you. Everybody gets to be free.

Review the checklist below, taken from page 71, then study the affirmations corresponding to each belief. Make these affirmations part of your daily routine. Say them often in the car, in the mirror, at work, or anytime you feel your negative beliefs surfacing.

If You Believe:	*Your Affirmation Is:*
Why are there so many bad drivers?	*I lovingly surround myself with wonderful drivers.*
People are so stupid.	*Everybody is doing the best they can, including me.*
I'm such a jerk.	*I love and approve of myself.*
I'd do it if I weren't so fat.	*I appreciate the wonder of my body.*
Those are the ugliest clothes I've ever seen.	*I love the uniqueness that people express in their clothing.*
They'll never be able to finish the job.	*I release the need to criticize others.*
I'm such a klutz.	*I become more proficient every day.*
The people around here are such slobs.	*I tidy up the rooms in my mind and this is reflected in everyone around me.*
My neighbors are so noisy.	*I release the need to be disturbed.*
Nobody asks me what I think.	*My opinions are valued.*
Can you believe that old car she drives?	*I lovingly support her choice of transportation.*
I hate his laugh.	*I rejoice in laughter whenever I hear it.*

POWER POINTS

1. We are each responsible for our experiences.

2. Every thought we think is creating our future.

3. Everyone is dealing with the damaging patterns of resentment, criticism, guilt, and self-hatred.

4. These are only thoughts and thoughts can be changed.

5. We need to release the past and forgive everyone, including ourselves.

6. Self-approval and self-acceptance in the "now" are the keys to positive changes.

7. The point of power is always in the present moment.

8

ADDICTIONS

*"No person, place, or thing has
any power over me. I am free."*

Addictions Checklist

- [ ] I want to feel better now.
- [ ] Smoking cigarettes reduces my
  stress.
- [ ] Having a lot of sex helps me to
  escape.
- [ ] I can't stop eating.
- [ ] Drinking makes me popular.
- [ ] I need perfection.
- [ ] I gamble too much.
- [ ] I need my tranquilizers.
- [ ] I can't stop buying things.
- [ ] I can't get away from abusive
  relationships.

*H*ow many of these sound like you? Let's take a closer look at this
behavior.

Addictive behavior is another way of saying, "I'm not good enough."
When we are caught in this type of behavior, we are trying to run away from

ourselves. We cannot be in touch with our feelings. Something that we are believing, saying, or doing is too painful for us to look at, so we overeat, drink, act out compulsive sexual behavior, take pills, spend money that we don't have, and create abusive love relationships.

There are 12-step programs that deal with most of these addictions, and they work well for thousands of people. We cannot hope to duplicate, in this chapter, what these programs have done for people with addictive behavior. I believe that we must first realize that there is a need in ourselves for the compulsive behavior. That need must be released before the behavior can be changed.

Loving and approving of yourself, trusting in the process of life, and feeling safe because you know the power of your own mind are extremely important issues when dealing with addictive behavior. My experiences with addicted persons have shown me that most share a deep self-hatred. They are very unforgiving of themselves. Day after day, they punish themselves. Why? Because somewhere along the line as children, they bought the idea that they were not good enough; they were bad and in need of punishment. Early childhood experiences that involve physical, emotional, or sexual abuse contribute to that self-hatred. Honesty, forgiveness, self-love, and a willingness to live in the truth can help to heal these early wounds and give the addictive person a reprieve from their behavior. I also find the addictive personality to be a fearful one. There is a great fear of letting go and trusting the life process. As long as we believe that the world is an unsafe place with people and situations waiting to "get" us—then that belief will be our reality.

Are you willing to let go of ideas and beliefs that don't support and nurture you? Then you are ready to continue our journey.

EXERCISE: *Release Your Addictions*

This is where the changes take place—right here and now in our own minds! Take some deep breaths, close your eyes, and think about the person, place, or thing that you are addicted to. Think of the insanity behind the addiction. You are trying to fix what you think is wrong inside of you by grabbing onto something that is outside of you. The point of power is in the present moment, and you can begin to make a shift today.

Once again, be willing to release the need. Say:

"I am willing to release the need for _____ in my life. I release it now and trust in the process of life to meet my needs."

Say it every morning in your daily meditation and prayers. You have taken another step to freedom.

EXERCISE: *Your Secret Addiction*

List 10 secrets that you have never shared with anyone regarding your addiction. If you are an overeater, maybe you have eaten out of a garbage can. If you are an alcoholic, you may have kept alcohol in the car so you could drink while driving. If you are a compulsive gambler, perhaps you put your family into jeopardy in order to borrow money to continue your addiction.

1. _____

2. _____

3. _____

4. _____

5. _____

6. _____

7. _____

8. _____

9. _____

10. _____

How do you feel now? Look at your "worst" secret. Visualize yourself at this period in your life and *love* that person. Tell them how much you love and forgive. Look into the mirror and say: "I forgive you and I love you exactly as you are." Breathe.

EXERCISE: *Ask Your Family*

Let's go back to our childhood for a moment and ask a few questions.

1. My mother always made me...

_____

_____

_____

_____

2. What I really wanted her to say was...

_____

_____

_____

_____

3. What my mother really didn't know was...

_____

_____

_____

_____

4. My father told me I shouldn't...

_____

_____

_____

_____

5. If my father only knew...

_____

_____

_____

_____

6. I wish I could have told my father...

_____

_____

_____

_____

7. Mother, I forgive you for...

_____

_____

_____

_____

8. Father, I forgive you for...

_____

_____

_____

_____

9. What would you still like to tell your parents about yourself? What is the unfinished business that you still have?

_____

_____

_____

_____

Many people come to me and say that they cannot enjoy today because of something that happened in the past. Holding on to the past *ONLY HURTS US*. We are refusing to live in the moment. The past is over and cannot be changed. This is the only moment we can experience.

EXERCISE: *Releasing the Past*

Let us now clean up the past in our minds. Release the emotional attachment to it. Allow the memories to be just memories.

If you remember what you wore at the age of 10, there is usually no attachment. It is just a memory.

That can be the same for all of the past events in our lives. As we let go, we become free to use all of our mental power to enjoy this moment and to create a bright future.

We don't have to keep punishing ourselves for the past.

1. List all of the things you are willing to let go of.

_____

_____

_____

_____

2. How willing are you to let go? Notice your reactions, and write them down.

_____

_____

_____

_____

3. What will you have to do to let these things go? How willing are you to do so?

_____

_____

_____

_____

_____

EXERCISE: *Self-Approval*

Since self-hatred plays such an important role in addictive behavior, we will now do one of my favorite and often-used exercises. I have given this exercise to thousands of people, and the results are phenomenal.

Every time that you think about your addiction for the next month, say over and over to yourself, "I APPROVE OF MYSELF."

Do this three or four hundred times a day. No, it's not too many times. When you are worrying, you will go over your problem at least that many times in a day. Let "I approve of myself" become a walking mantra, something that you say over and over to yourself, almost nonstop.

Saying "I approve of myself" is guaranteed to bring up everything in your consciousness that is in opposition. When a negative thought like, "How can you approve of yourself—you spent all of your money" or "You just ate two pieces of cake" or "You'll never amount to anything," or whatever your negative babble may be, *this* is the time to take mental control. Give it no importance. Just see the thought for what it is, another way to keep you stuck in the past. Gently say to this thought, "Thank you for sharing. I let you go, I approve of myself." These thoughts of resistance will have no power over you unless you choose to believe them.

Refer to the checklist on the next page, taken from page 81. Find the affirmation corresponding to each belief. Make these affirmations part of your daily schedule. Say them at work, in the car, or while brushing your teeth in the morning.

If You Believe:	*Your Affirmation Is:*
I want to feel better now.	*I am at peace.*
Smoking cigarettes reduces my stress.	*I release my stress with ease.*
Having a lot of sex helps me to escape.	*I have the power, strength, and knowledge to handle everything in my life.*
I can't stop eating.	*Love surrounds me and protects me and nourishes me.*
Drinking makes me popular.	*I radiate acceptance and I am deeply loved by others.*
I need perfection.	*I allow and welcome change.*
I gamble too much.	*I am open to the wisdom within.*
I need my tranquilizers.	*I relax into the flow of life and let life provide all that I need easily and comfortably.*
I can't stop buying things.	*I am willing to create new thoughts about myself and my life.*
I can't get away from abusive relationships.	*I am powerful and capable. I love and appreciate all of myself.*

"I give myself permission to change."

POWER POINTS

1. We are each responsible for our experiences.

2. Every thought we think is creating our future.

3. Everyone is dealing with the damaging patterns of resentment, criticism, guilt, and self-hatred.

4. These are only thoughts and thoughts can be changed.

5. We need to release the past and forgive everyone, including ourselves.

6. Self-approval and self-acceptance in the "now" are the keys to positive changes.

7. The point of power is always in the present moment.

FORGIVENESS

"I am forgiven and I am free."

Forgiveness Checklist

☐ I'll never forgive them.
☐ What they did was unforgivable.
☐ They ruined my life.
☐ They did it on purpose.
☐ I was so little, and they hurt me so much.
☐ They have to apologize first.
☐ My resentment keeps me safe.
☐ Only weak people forgive.
☐ I'm right and they are wrong.
☐ It's all my parents' fault.
☐ I don't have to forgive anyone.

Do you resonate to several of these statements? Forgiveness is a difficult area for most of us.

We all need to do forgiveness work. Anyone who has a problem with loving themselves is stuck in this area. Forgiveness opens our hearts to self-love.

Many of us carry grudges for years and years. We feel self-righteous because of what *they* did to us. I call this being stuck in the prison of self-righteous resentment. We get to be right. We never get to be happy.

I can hear you saying, "But you don't know what they did to me, it's unforgivable." Being unwilling to forgive is a terrible thing to do to ourselves. Bitterness is like swallowing a teaspoon of poison every day. It accumulates and harms us. It is impossible to be healthy and free when we keep ourselves bound to the past. The incident is long over. Yes, they did not behave well. However, it is over. Sometimes we feel that if we forgive them, then we are saying that what they did to us was okay.

One of our biggest spiritual lessons is to understand that "everyone" is doing the best they can at any given moment. People can only do so much with the understanding, awareness, and knowledge that they have. Invariably, anyone who mistreats someone was mistreated as a child. The greater the violence, the greater their own inner pain. This is not to condone poor behavior. However, for our own spiritual growth, we must be aware of their pain.

The incident is over. Perhaps long over. Let it go. Allow yourself to be free. Come out of prison and step into the sunshine of life. If the incident is still going on, then ask yourself why you think so little of yourself that you still put up with it. Why do you stay in such a situation? The purpose of this book is to help you raise your self-esteem to such a level that you only allow loving experiences in your life. Don't waste time trying to "get even." It doesn't work. What we give out always comes back to us. So let's drop the past and work on loving ourselves in the now. Then we shall have a wonderful future.

That person who is the hardest to forgive is the one who can teach you the greatest lessons. When you love yourself enough to rise above the old situation, then understanding and forgiveness will be easy. And you will be free. Does freedom frighten you? Does it feel safer to be stuck in your old resentment and bitterness?

MIRROR WORK

Time to go back to our friend, the mirror. Look into your eyes and say with feeling, "I am willing to forgive!" Repeat this several times.

What are you feeling? Do you feel stubborn and stuck? Or, do you feel open and willing?

Just notice your feelings. Don't judge them. Breathe deeply a few times and repeat the exercise. Does it feel any different?

EXERCISE: *Family Attitudes*

1. Was your mother a forgiving person?

_____

_____

_____

_____

2. Was your father a forgiving person?

_____

_____

_____

_____

3. Was bitterness a family way of handling hurts?

_____

_____

_____

_____

4. How did your mother get even?

_____

_____

_____

_____

5. How did your father get even?

_____

_____

_____

_____

6. How do you get even?

_____

_____

_____

_____

7. Do you feel good when you get revenge?

_____

_____

_____

_____

8. Why?

_____

_____

_____

_____

An interesting phenomenon is that when we do our own forgiveness work, other people often respond to it. It is not necessary to go to the person involved and tell them that you forgive them. Sometimes you want to do this. You do not have to. The major work of forgiveness is done in your own heart.

Forgiveness is seldom for "them." It is for us. The person you need to forgive may even be dead.

I have heard from many people that when they have truly forgiven, a month or two later, they may receive a phone call or a letter from the other person, asking to be forgiven. This seems to be particularly true for forgiveness done in front of a mirror. As you do this exercise, notice how deep your feelings might be.

MIRROR WORK

Mirror work is often uncomfortable and something we want to run from. If you are standing in the bathroom doing mirror work, it is far too easy to run out the door. I believe that you receive the most benefits if you sit in front of a mirror. I like to use the big dressing mirror on the back of the bedroom door. I settle in with a box of tissues. My dog often sits beside me to comfort me as I do mirror work.

Give yourself time to do this exercise, or you can do it over and over. We all have lots of people to forgive. Sit in front of your mirror. Close your eyes and breathe deeply several times. Think of the many people who have hurt you in your life. Let them pass through your mind. Now open your eyes and begin talking to one of them.

Say something like, "You have hurt me deeply. However, I won't stay stuck in the past any longer. I am willing to forgive you." Take a breath and say, "I forgive you and I set you free." Breathe again and say, "You are free and I am free."

Notice how you feel. You may feel resistance, or you may feel clear. If you feel resistance, just breathe and say, "I am willing to release all resistance."

This may be a day when you can forgive several people. It may be a day when you can forgive only one. It doesn't matter. However you are doing this exercise is perfect for you. Forgiveness can be like peeling away the layers of an onion. If there are too many tears, put the onion away for a day. You can always come back and peel another layer. Acknowledge yourself for being willing to even begin this exercise.

As you continue to do this exercise, today or another day, expand your list of those to forgive. Remember:

Family
Teachers
Kids at school
Lovers
Friends
The work environment
Government agencies or figures

Church personnel
Hospital personnel
Other authority figures
God
Myself

Most of all, forgive yourself. Stop being hard on yourself. Self-punishment isn't necessary. You were doing the very best you could.

Sit in front of the mirror once again with your list. Say to each person on your list, "I forgive you for _____." Breathe. "I forgive you and I set you free."

Continue to go down your list, if you feel free from anger with a person, cross them off. If you are not free of anger, put them aside and come back to the work later.

As you continue to do this exercise, you will find burdens melting off your shoulders. You may be surprised to notice how much old baggage you have been carrying. Be gentle with yourself as you go through the cleansing process.

MAKE A LIST

Put on some soft music—something that will make you feel relaxed and peaceful. Now take a pad and pen, and let your mind drift. Go back into the past, and think of all the things that you are angry with yourself over. Write them down. Write them all down. You may discover that you have never forgiven yourself for wetting your pants and being embarrassed in the first grade. What a long time to carry *that* burden!

Sometimes it is easier to forgive others than to forgive ourselves. We are often hard on ourselves, and demand perfection. Any mistakes we make are severely punished. It's time to go beyond that old attitude.

Mistakes are the way we learn. If we were perfect, there wouldn't be anything to learn. We wouldn't need to be on the planet. Being "perfect" will not even get your parents' love and approval—it will only make you feel "wrong" and not good enough. Lighten up and stop treating yourself that way.

Forgive yourself. Let it go. Give yourself the space to be spontaneous and free. There is no need for shame and guilt.

Remember how wonderful it was to run free when you were a child.

Go outside to a beach, a park, or even an empty lot, and let yourself run. Do not jog. Run wild and free—turn somersaults—skip—and laugh while you are doing it! Take your inner child with you and have some fun. So what if someone sees you? This is for your freedom!

Review the checklist below, taken from page 91. Find the corresponding affirmation below for each negative belief.

If You Believe:	*Your Affirmation Is:*
I'll never forgive them.	*This is a new moment. I am free to let go.*
They don't deserve to be forgiven.	*I forgive whether they deserve it or not.*
What they did to me was unforgivable.	*I am willing to go beyond my own limitations.*
They ruined my life.	*I take responsibility for my own life. I am free.*
They did it on purpose.	*They were doing the best they could with the knowledge, understanding, and awareness that they had at the time.*
I was so little and they hurt me so much.	*I am grown up now and I take loving care of my inner child.*
They have to apologize first.	*My spiritual growth is not dependent on others.*
My resentment keeps me safe.	*I release myself from prison. I am safe and free.*
Only weak people forgive.	*It is strong to forgive and let go.*
I'm right and they are wrong.	*There is no right or wrong. I move beyond my judgment.*
It's all my parents' fault.	*My parents treated me the way they had been treated. I forgive them and their parents, too.*
I don't have to forgive anyone.	*I refuse to limit myself. I am always willing to take the next step.*

"I give myself permission to let go."

POWER POINTS

1. We are each responsible for our experiences.

2. Every thought we think is creating our future.

3. Everyone is dealing with the damaging patterns of resentment, criticism, guilt, and self-hatred.

4. These are only thoughts and thoughts can be changed.

5. We need to release the past and forgive everyone, including ourselves.

6. Self-approval and self-acceptance in the "now" are the keys to positive changes.

7. The point of power is always in the present moment.

10

WORK

"It is a joy to express my creativity and be appreciated."

Work Checklist

- [ ] I hate my job.
- [ ] My job is too stressful.
- [ ] No one appreciates me at work.
- [ ] I always get dead-end jobs.
- [ ] My boss is abusive.
- [ ] Everyone expects too much of me.
- [ ] My co-workers drive me crazy.
- [ ] My job offers no creativity.
- [ ] I'll never be successful.
- [ ] There is no chance for advancement.
- [ ] My job doesn't pay well.

How many of these sound like you? Let's explore your thinking in the work area.

Our jobs and the work that we do are a reflection of our own self-worth and our value to the world. On one level, work is an exchange of time and services for money. As long as we are doing an honest day's work, our self-esteem can be in order.

However, the *kind* of work we do is important to us because we are unique individuals. We want to feel that we are making a contribution to the world. We need to use our own talents, intelligence, and creative ability.

There are problems that can occur in the workplace, though. You may not get along with your boss or your co-workers. You may not feel appreciated or recognized for the work that you do. Promotional opportunities or a specific job may elude you.

Remember that whatever position you may find yourself in...your thinking got you there. The people around you are only mirroring what *you* believe you deserve.

Thoughts can be changed. Situations can be changed as well. That boss that we find intolerable could become our champion. That dead-end position with no hope of advancement may open up to a new career full of possibilities. The co-worker who is so annoying might turn out to be, if not a friend, at least someone who is easier to get along with. The salary that we find insufficient can increase in the twinkle of an eye. We could find a wonderful new job.

There are an infinite number of channels if we can change *our* thinking. Let's open ourselves up to them. We must accept in consciousness that abundance and fulfillment can come from anywhere. The change may be small at first, such as an added assignment from your boss in which you could demonstrate your intelligence and creativity. You may treat a co-worker as if they were not the enemy and as a result, experience a notable change in behavior. Whatever the change may be, accept and rejoice in it. You are not alone. You *are* the change. The power that created you has given *you* the power to create your own experiences!

EXERCISE: *Center Yourself*

Let's take a moment to center ourselves. Take your right hand and place it over your lower stomach area. Think of this area as the center of your being. Breathe. Look into your mirror again and say, "I am willing to release the need to be so unhappy at work." Say it two more times. Each time say it a different way. You want to increase your commitment to change.

EXERCISE: *Describe the People in Your Life*

Use 10 adjectives to describe your:

	Boss	Co-workers	Position
1.			
2.			
3.			
4.			
5.			
6.			
7.			
8.			
9.			
10.			

EXERCISE: *Think About Your Work Life*

1. If you could become anything, what would you be?

_____

_____

_____

_____

2. If you could have any job that you wanted, what would it be?

_____

_____

_____

_____

3. What would you like to change about your present job?

_____

_____

_____

_____

4. How would you change your employer?

_____

_____

_____

_____

5. Do you work in a pleasant environment?

_____

_____

_____

_____

6. Whom do you need to forgive the most at work?

_____

_____

_____

_____

MIRROR WORK

Sit in front of your mirror. Breathe deeply. Center yourself. Now talk to the person at work you are most angry with. Tell them why you are angry. Tell them how much they have hurt you or threatened you, or violated your space and boundaries. Tell them everything—don't hold back! Tell them the kind of behavior you want from them in the future. Tell them that you forgive them for not being who you wanted them to be.

Take a breath. Ask them to give you respect and offer the same to them. Affirm that you can both have a harmonious working relationship.

Blessing With Love

Blessing with love is a powerful tool to use in any work environment. Send it ahead of you before you arrive. Bless every person. place, or thing there with love. If you have a problem with a co-worker, a boss, a supplier, or even the temperature, bless it with love. Affirm that you and the person or situation are in agreement and in perfect harmony.

"I am in perfect harmony with my work environment and everyone in it."

"I always work in harmonious surroundings."

"I honor and respect each person, and they, in turn, honor and respect me."

"I bless this situation with love, and know that it works out the best for everyone concerned."

"I bless you with love and release you to your highest good."

"I bless this job and release it to someone who will love it, and I am free to accept a wonderful new opportunity."

Select or adapt one of these affirmations to fit a situation in your workplace, and repeat it over and over." Every time the person or situation comes into mind, repeat the affirmation. Eliminate the negative energy in your mind regarding this situation. You can, just by thinking, change the experience.

EXERCISE: *Self-Worth in Your Job*

Let's examine your feelings of self-worth in the area of employment. After answering the following questions, write an affirmation (in the present tense).

1. **Do I feel worthy of having a good job?**

   Example:
   Sometimes I feel worthy. But when I don't I feel like hiding.

YOUR EXAMPLE:

_____

_____

_____

_____

Sample Affirmation:
I am totally adequate for all situations.

YOUR AFFIRMATION:

_____

_____

_____

_____

2. What do I fear most in this area?

Example:
That my employer will find out that I am no good, fire me, and I won't find another job.

YOUR EXAMPLE:

_____

_____

_____

_____

Sample Affirmation:
I center myself in safety and accept the perfection of my life. All is well.

YOUR AFFIRMATION:

_____

_____

_____

_____

3. What am I "getting" from this belief?

Example:
I people-please at work, and turn my employer into a parent.

YOUR EXAMPLE:

_____

_____

_____

_____

Sample Affirmation:
It is my mind that creates my experiences. I am unlimited in my ability to create the good in my life.

YOUR AFFIRMATION:

_____

_____

_____

_____

4. What do I fear would happen if I let go of this belief?

Example:
I would have to grow up.
I would have to be responsible.

YOUR EXAMPLE:

_____

_____

_____

_____

Sample Affirmation:
I know that I am worthwhile. It is safe for me to succeed. Life loves me.
YOUR AFFIRMATION:

_____

_____

_____

_____

VISUALIZATION

What would the perfect job be? Take a moment to see yourself in that job. See yourself in the environment, see your co-workers, and feel what it would be like to do work that was completely fulfilling, while you earn a good salary. Hold that vision for yourself and know that it has been completed in consciousness.

Refer to the checklist on the next page, taken from page 99. Find the affirmation corresponding to each belief. Make these affirmations part of your daily schedule. Say them at work, in the car, or when brushing your teeth in the morning.

If You Believe:	*Your Affirmation Is:*
My job is too stressful.	*I am always relaxed at work.*
No one appreciates me at work.	*My work is recognized by everyone.*
I always get dead-end jobs.	*I turn every experience into an opportunity.*
My boss is abusive.	*I respect myself and so do others.*
Everyone expects too much of me.	*I am in the perfect place, and I am safe at all times.*
My co-workers drive me crazy.	*I see the best in everyone and help them to bring out their most joyous qualities.*
My job offers no creativity.	*My thoughts are creative.*
I'll never be successful.	*Everything I touch is a success.*
There is no chance for advancement.	*New doors are opening all the time.*
My job doesn't pay well.	*I am open and receptive to new avenues of income.*

"I give myself permission to be creatively fulfilled."

POWER POINTS

1. We are each responsible for our experiences.

2. Every thought we think is creating our future.

3. Everyone is dealing with the damaging patterns of resentment, criticism, guilt, and self-hatred.

4. These are only thoughts and thoughts can be changed.

5. We need to release the past and forgive everyone, including ourselves.

6. Self-approval and self-acceptance in the "now" are the keys to positive changes.

7. The point of power is always in the present moment.

11

MONEY AND PROSPERITY

"Infinite prosperity is mine to share; I am blessed."

Money and Prosperity Checklist

- ☐ I can't save money.
- ☐ I don't earn enough.
- ☐ My credit rating is bad.
- ☐ Money slips through my fingers.
- ☐ Everything is so expensive.
- ☐ Why does everyone else have money?
- ☐ I can't pay my bills.
- ☐ Bankruptcy is around the corner.
- ☐ I can't save for retirement.
- ☐ I can't let go of money.

*H*ow many of these sound like you? If you have checked off three or more, work on your money issues.

What do you believe about money? Do you believe that there is enough? Do you attach your self-worth to it? Do you think that it will bring your heart's desire? Are you friends with money or is it an enemy? Having more money is not enough. We need to learn how to deserve and *enjoy* the money that we have.

Large amounts of money do not guarantee prosperity. People who have a lot of money can be engulfed in poverty consciousness. They can be more fearful about not having money than someone who lives on the streets. The ability to enjoy their money and to live in a world of abundance may elude them. Socrates, the great philosopher, once said that "contentment is natural wealth, luxury is artificial poverty."

As I have said many times, your prosperity consciousness is not dependent upon money; your flow of money is dependent upon your prosperity consciousness.

Our pursuit of money *must* contribute to the quality of our lives. If it does not, that is, if we hate what we do in order to get money, then money will be useless. Prosperity involves the *quality* of our lives as well as any amount of money that we possess.

Prosperity is not defined by money alone; it encompasses time, love, success, joy, comfort, beauty, and wisdom. For example, you can be poor with respect to time. If you feel rushed, pressured, and harried, then your time is steeped in poverty. But, if you feel you have all of the time you need to finish any task at hand, and you are confident that you can finish any job, then you are prosperous when it comes to time.

Or what about success? Do you feel that it's beyond your reach and completely unattainable? Or do you feel that you can be a success in your own right? If you do, then you are rich with respect to success.

Know that whatever your beliefs are, they can be changed in *this* moment. The power that created you has given *you* the power to create your own experiences. You can change!

MIRROR WORK

Stand up with your arms outstretched and say, "I am open and receptive to all good." How does that feel?

Now, look into the mirror and say it again with more feeling.

What kinds of feelings come up for you? Does it feel liberating and joyous? Or do you feel like hiding?

Breathe deeply—say again—"I am open and receptive to _____ _____ (you fill in the blank). Do this exercise every morning. It is a wonderfully symbolic gesture that may increase your prosperity consciousness and bring more good into your life.

EXERCISE: *Your Feelings About Money*

Let's examine your feelings of self-worth in this area. Answer the following questions as best you can.

1. Go back to the mirror. Look into your eyes and say: "My biggest fear about money is _____." Write down your answer.

_____

_____

_____

_____

2. What did you learn about money as a child?

_____

_____

_____

_____

3. Did your parents grow up during the Depression era? What were their thoughts about money?

_____

_____

_____

_____

4. How were finances handled in your family?

_____

_____

_____

_____

5. How do you handle money now?

_____

_____

_____

_____

6. What would you like to change about your money consciousness?

_____

_____

_____

_____

EXERCISE: *Your Money Consciousness*

Let's examine the feelings of self-worth in the money area. Answer the following questions as best you can. After each negative belief, construct a positive affirmation in the present tense to take its place.

1. Do I feel worthy of having and enjoying money?

Example:
Not really. I get rid of money as soon as I get it.

YOUR EXAMPLE:

_____

_____

_____

_____

Sample Affirmation:
I bless the money I have. It is safe to save money and let my money work for me.

YOUR AFFIRMATION:

_____

_____

_____

_____

2. **What is my greatest fear regarding money?**

   Example:
   I am afraid that I'll always be broke.

   YOUR EXAMPLE:

   _____

   _____

   _____

   _____

   Sample Affirmation:
   I now accept limitless abundance from a limitless universe.

   YOUR AFFIRMATION:

   _____

   _____

   _____

   _____

3. **What am I "getting" from this belief?**

   Example:
   I stay poor and I get to be taken care of by others.

YOUR EXAMPLE:

_____

_____

_____

_____

Sample Affirmation:
I claim my own power and lovingly create my own reality. I trust the process of life.

YOUR AFFIRMATION:

_____

_____

_____

_____

4. What do I fear would happen to me if I let go of this belief?

Example:
No one would love and take care of me.

YOUR EXAMPLE:

_____

_____

_____

_____

Sample Affirmation:
I am safe in the Universe, and all life loves and supports me.

YOUR AFFIRMATION:

_____

_____

_____

_____

_____

EXERCISE: *Your Use of Money*

Write down three ways in which you criticize your use of money. Maybe you are constantly in debt, you can't save money, or you cannot enjoy your money.

Think of one way in each of these instances where you have not *acted out the undesired behavior.*

Examples:

I Criticize Myself for: *compulsively spending money and being in constant debt. I can't seem to hold down my spending.*

I Praise Myself for: *paying the rent on time today. It is the first of the month, and I paid the rent.*

I Criticize Myself for: *saving every penny that I make. I can't let go of my money.*

I Praise Myself for: *buying a shirt that was not on sale. I let myself have what I really wanted today.*

1. I criticize myself for:

_____

_____

_____

_____

I praise myself for:

_____

_____

_____

_____

2. I criticize myself for:

_____

_____

_____

_____

I praise myself for:

_____

_____

_____

_____

3. I criticize myself for:

_____

_____

_____

_____

I praise myself for:

_____

_____

_____

_____

VISUALIZATION-1

Place your hand over your heart, take a few deep breaths, and relax. See yourself acting out your worst scenario with money. Perhaps you borrowed money that you couldn't return, bought something you knew you could not afford, or declared bankruptcy. See yourself acting out the behavior—*love that person*. Know that you were doing the very best you could with the knowledge understanding, and capability that you had. *Love that person*. See yourself acting out behavior that might embarrass you today and *love that person*.

VISUALIZATION-2

What would it be like to have all of the things you've always wanted? What would they look like? Where would you go? What would you do? Feel it. Enjoy it. Be creative and HAVE FUN.

Refer to the checklist on the next page, taken from page 109. Find the affirmation corresponding to each belief. Make these affirmations part of your daily schedule. Say them at work, in the car, in the mirror, or while brushing your teeth in the morning.

If You Believe:	*Your Affirmation Is:*
I can't save money.	*I always have a savings account.*
I don't earn enough money.	*My income is constantly increasing.*
My credit rating is bad.	*My credit rating is getting better all the time.*
Money slips through my fingers.	*I spend money wisely.*
Everything is so expensive.	*I always have as much as I need.*
Why does everyone else have money?	*I have as much money as I can accept.*
I can't pay my bills.	*I bless all of my bills. I pay them on time.*
Bankruptcy is around the corner.	*I am financially solvent.*
I can't save for retirement.	*I am providing for my retirement.*
I can't let go of money.	*I enjoy every penny that I spend.*

"I give myself permission to prosper."

POWER POINTS

1. We are each responsible for our experiences.

2. Every thought we think is creating our future.

3. Everyone is dealing with the damaging patterns of resentment, criticism, guilt, and self-hatred.

4. These are only thoughts and thoughts can be changed.

5. We need to release the past and forgive everyone, including ourselves.

6. Self-approval and self-acceptance in the "now" are the keys to positive changes.

7. The point of power is always in the present moment.

12

FRIENDS

"I am a friend to myself."

Friendship Checklist

- ☐ My friends don't support me.
- ☐ Everyone is so judgmental.
- ☐ Nobody sees it my way.
- ☐ My boundaries are not respected.
- ☐ I can't keep friends for too long.
- ☐ I can't let my friends really know me.
- ☐ I give my friends advice for their own good.
- ☐ I don't know how to be a friend.
- ☐ I don't know how to ask for help from my friends.
- ☐ I don't know how to tell a friend "no."

How many of these sound like you? Let's see if we can improve the quality of your friendships.

Friendships can be our most enduring and important relationships. We can live without lovers or spouses. We can live without our primary families, but most of us cannot live happily without friends. I believe that we choose our parents before we are born into this planet, but we choose our friends on a more conscious level.

Ralph Waldo Emerson, the great American philosopher and writer, wrote an essay on friendship, calling it the "nectar of the gods." He explained that in romantic relationships, one person is always trying to change the other, but friends can stand back and look at one another with appreciation and respect.

Friends can be an extension or a substitute for the nuclear family. There is a great need in most of us to share life experiences with others. Not only do we learn more about others when we engage in friendship, but we can also learn more about ourselves. These relationships are mirrors of our self-worth and esteem. They afford us the perfect opportunity to look at ourselves, and the areas where we might need to grow.

When the bond between friends becomes strained, we can look to the negative messages of childhood. It may be time for mental housecleaning. Cleaning the mental house after a lifetime of negative messages is a bit like going on a good nutritional program after a lifetime of eating junk foods. As you change your diet, the body will throw off a toxic residue, and you may feel worse for a day or two.

So it is when you make a decision to change mental thought patterns. Your circumstances may worsen for a while. But remember! You may have to dig through a lot of dry weed to get to the rich soil below. But you can do it! I know you can!

EXERCISE: *Your Friendships*

In the space provided below, write out the following affirmation three times:

"I am willing to release the pattern in me that creates troubled friendships."

_____

_____

_____

1. What were your first childhood friendships like?

_____

_____

_____

_____

2. **How are your friendships today like those childhood friendships?**

   Example:
   I always allowed myself to be bossed around by my friends. I still look for friends who are bossy.

   _____

   _____

   _____

   _____

3. **What did you learn about friendships from your parents?**

   _____

   _____

   _____

   _____

4. **What kind of friends did your parents have?**

   _____

   _____

   _____

   _____

5. **What kind of friends would you like to have in the future? Be specific.**

   _____

   _____

   _____

   _____

   _____

Let's examine our self-worth in the area of friendships. Answer each of the following questions below. After each answer write a positive affirmation (in the present tense) to replace the old belief.

1. Do I feel worthy in the area of friendship?

Example:
No. Why would anyone want to be around me?

YOUR EXAMPLE:

_____

_____

_____

_____

Sample Affirmation:
I love and accept myself, and I am a magnet for friends.

YOUR AFFIRMATION:

_____

_____

_____

_____

2. What do I fear most in the area of friendships?

Example:
I am afraid of betrayal. I don't feel I can trust anyone.

YOUR EXAMPLE:

_____

_____

_____

_____

Sample Affirmation:
I trust myself, I trust life, and I trust my friends.

YOUR AFFIRMATION:

_____

_____

_____

_____

3. What am I "getting" from this belief?

Example:
I get to be judgmental. I wait for my friends to make one false move so that I can make them wrong.

YOUR EXAMPLE:

_____

_____

_____

_____

Sample Affirmation:
All of my friendships are successful. I am a loving and nurturing friend.

YOUR AFFIRMATION:

_____

_____

_____

_____

4. What do I fear would happen if I let go of this belief?

Example:
I would lose control. I would have to let people really know me.

YOUR EXAMPLE:

_____

_____

_____

_____

Sample Affirmation:
Loving others is easy when I love and accept myself.

YOUR AFFIRMATION:

_____

_____

_____

_____

If we are all responsible for the events in our lives, then there is no one to blame. Whatever is happening "out there" is only a reflection of our own inner thinking.

EXERCISE: *Think About Your Friends*

Think of three events in your life in which you feel you were mistreated or abused by friends. Perhaps a friend betrayed a confidence, or abandoned you in time of need. Maybe they interfered with a spouse or mate.

In each case, name the event and write down some of the thoughts IN YOUR MIND that preceded each event.

Example:

When I was 16 years old, my best friend Susie turned on me and started to spread vicious rumors. When I tried to confront her, she lied to me. I was friendless for my whole senior year.

My deepest thoughts were: *I did not deserve friends. I was drawn to my friend Susie because she was cold and judgmental. I was used to being judged and criticized.*

1. The event:

_____

_____

_____

_____

   My deepest thoughts were:

_____

_____

_____

_____

2. The event:

_____

_____

_____

_____

   My deepest thoughts were:

_____

_____

_____

_____

3. The event:

_____

_____

_____

_____

My deepest thoughts were:

_____

_____

_____

_____

EXERCISE: *The Support of Your Friends*

Think of three events in your life where you were supported by friends. Perhaps a good friend stood up for you, or gave you money when you needed it. Maybe they helped you to resolve a difficult situation.

In each case, name the event and write down some of the thoughts "in your mind" that preceded each event.

Example:

I will always remember Helen. When people at my first job were making fun of me because I said something stupid at a meeting, Helen stood beside me. She helped me through my embarrassment and saved my job.

My deepest thoughts were: *Even if I make a mistake, someone will always help me through. I deserve to be supported. Women support me.*

1. The event:

_____

_____

_____

_____

My deepest thoughts were:

_____

_____

_____

_____

2. The event:

_____

_____

_____

_____

My deepest thoughts were:

_____

_____

_____

_____

3. The event:

_____

_____

_____

_____

My deepest thoughts were:

_____

_____

_____

_____

PRAISE AND ACKNOWLEDGEMENT

Which friends do I need to acknowledge?
Take a moment to visualize them. Look at that person in the eye and say:
"I thank you and bless you with love for being there for me when I needed you. May your life be filled with joy."

ANGER-RELEASING VISUALIZATION

Which friends do you need to forgive?
Take a moment to visualize them. Now look that person in the eye and say, "I forgive you for not acting the way I wanted you to. I forgive you and I set you free."

Read the list of negative beliefs on the next page, taken from page 121. Find the corresponding affirmations next to them. Make these affirmations part of your daily prayer. Say them in the car, at work, or in the bathroom mirror each morning.

If You Believe:	Your Affirmation Is:
My friends don't support me.	*My friends are loving and supportive.*
Everyone is so judgmental.	*I am safe in the world and all life loves and supports me.*
Nobody sees it my way.	*I am open and receptive to all points of view.*
My boundaries are not respected.	*I respect others and they respect me.*
I can't keep friends for too long.	*My love and acceptance of others creates lasting friendships.*
I can't let my friends really know me.	*It is safe for me to be open.*
I give my friends advice for their own good.	*My friends and I have total freedom to be ourselves.*
I don't know how to be a friend.	*I trust my inner wisdom to guide me.*
I don't know how to ask for help from my friends.	*It is safe to ask for what I want.*
I don't know how to tell an old friend "no."	*I move beyond limitations and express myself freely.*

"I give myself permission to be a friend."

POWER POINTS

1. We are each responsible for our experiences.

2. Every thought we think is creating our future.

3. Everyone is dealing with the damaging patterns of resentment, criticism, guilt, and self-hatred.

4. These are only thoughts and thoughts can be changed.

5. We need to release the past and forgive everyone, including ourselves.

6. Self-approval and self-acceptance in the "now" are the keys to positive changes.

7. The point of power is always in the present moment.

13

SEXUALITY

"I am at peace with my own sexuality."

Sexuality Checklist

- ☐ I am afraid of sex.
- ☐ Sex is dirty.
- ☐ Genitals frighten me.
- ☐ I don't get what I want.
- ☐ I am the wrong size or shape.
- ☐ I am ashamed of my sexuality.
- ☐ I can't ask for what I want.
- ☐ God doesn't want me to be sexual.
- ☐ My partner won't like my body.
- ☐ I am afraid of dis-ease.
- ☐ I am not good enough.
- ☐ Sex is painful.

*H*ow many of these sound like you? If you have checked off three or more, concentrate on this area.

Sex is a difficult area for a lot of people. Many complain that they are getting too much or too little. Sex threatens them, motivates them, maddens them, and offers escape. It can be tender, loving, joyful, painful, explosive, wondrous, fulfilling, or humiliating.

People often equate sex with love, or they need to be in love to have sex. Many of us grew up believing that sex was sinful unless we were married, or that sex was for procreation and not for pleasure. Some people have rebelled against this concept and feel that sex has nothing to do with love.

Most of our beliefs about sex can be traced to our childhood and our ideas about God and religion. Most of us were raised with the idea of what I call "Mama's God," which is what your mother taught you about God when you were very little. It is often the image of God as an old man with a beard. This old man sits on a cloud and stares at people's genitals, waiting to catch someone sinning.

Think for a moment about the vastness of the universe. How perfect it all is! Think about the level of intelligence that created it. I have a difficult time believing that this same divine intelligence could resemble a judgmental old man watching *my* genitals.

When we were babies, we knew how perfect our bodies were, and we loved our sexuality. Babies are never ashamed of themselves. *No baby ever measures its hips to find its self-worth.*

We must let go of images and beliefs that do not nourish and support us. I believe that the sexual revolution, which occurred in the late '60s, was a good thing in many ways. We were freed from Victorian ideas and hypocrisy. Of course, when people are freed from oppression, they go wild for a while. Eventually, the pendulum will swing back until it reaches a balance point—neither too wild nor too oppressed. I believe that sex is meant to be a joyful, loving act, and as long as our hearts are open, and we really care about ourselves, we will not harm ourselves or others. However, sex can be another form of abuse and express low self-worth. If we constantly need a new partner to make us feel worthy, or allow infidelity to be a way of life, we need to examine our thinking.

VISUALIZATION

Before you answer the following questions, lie down or sit in a comfortable position. Close your eyes and put both hands over your heart. Picture a stream of brilliant white light entering your heart. Focus on the vision of light and say out loud: "I am willing to let the love in." Feel the energy flowing into your heart. After a few minutes, repeat this several times, open your eyes and say: "All is well."

Answer the following questions as best you can.

1. What did you learn about sex as a child?

_____

_____

_____

_____

2. What did your parents teach you about the human body? Was it beautiful, or was it something to be ashamed of?

_____

_____

_____

_____

3. What did teachers or your church say about sex? Was it a sin to be punished for?

_____

_____

_____

_____

4. What were your genitals called? Or were they just something "down there?"

_____

_____

_____

_____

5. Do you think that your parents had a fulfilling sex life?

_____

_____

_____

_____

6. How are your ideas about sex similar to those of your parents?

_____

_____

_____

_____

7. How are they different?

_____

_____

_____

_____

8. What did God "think" about sex when you were little?

_____

_____

_____

_____

9. Do you equate sex with love?

_____

_____

_____

_____

10. How do you feel during the sex act itself? Do you feel loving and tender? Do you feel powerful? Are you guilty?

_____

_____

_____

_____

11. Have you ever abused yourself or another sexually?

_____

_____

_____

_____

12. Have you ever been abused sexually?

_____

_____

_____

_____

13. If you could change anything about sex in your life, what would it be?

_____

_____

_____

_____

MIRROR WORK

Now look in the mirror, into your own eyes, and say: "I am willing to love my body and my sexuality." Say it three times, with more meaning and feeling each time. Then, answer these questions.

1. What are your most negative thoughts about your body?

_____

_____

_____

_____

2. Where did these thoughts come from?

_____

_____

_____

3. Are you willing to release them?   ☐ Yes   ☐ No

Now, let's examine the issue of self-worth. Answer the questions on the next page, and after each one, create a corresponding affirmation.

1. **Do I deserve to enjoy my sexuality?**

   Example:
   No. I hate the shape of my body. I want to hurry up and get sex over with.
   I feel ugly.

   YOUR EXAMPLE:

   _____

   _____

   _____

   _____

   Sample Affirmation:
   *I love and appreciate my beautiful body. It is the perfect size and shape for
   me. I rejoice in my sexuality.*

   YOUR AFFIRMATION:

   _____

   _____

   _____

   _____

2. **What do I fear most about my sexuality?**

   Example:
   I fear being laughed at. I am afraid of doing it wrong, or not knowing
   what to do. I am afraid of feeling dirty.

   YOUR EXAMPLE:

   _____

   _____

   _____

   _____

   Sample Affirmation:
   My sexuality is a wonderful gift. I love being creative. I am safe.

YOUR AFFIRMATION:

_____

_____

_____

_____

3. What am I "getting" from this belief?

Example:
I get protection. I get to feel safe. I don't want anyone coming close to me with their genitals. Genitals scare me.

YOUR EXAMPLE:

_____

_____

_____

_____

Sample Affirmation:
It is safe to be myself. I love all of my body. I trust in the life process to keep me safe.

YOUR AFFIRMATION:

_____

_____

_____

_____

4. What do I fear would happen if I let go of this belief?

Example:
I am afraid that I would lose control. I am afraid that I would get lost. There would be no more "me."

YOUR EXAMPLE:

_____

_____

_____

_____

Sample Affirmation:
I am safe to be me in all situations. I rejoice in my individuality.

YOUR AFFIRMATION:

_____

_____

_____

_____

Review the belief checklist on the next page, taken from page 133, then study the affirmations corresponding to each belief. Make these affirmations part of your daily routine. Say them often in the car, at work, or any time you feel your negative beliefs surfacing.

If You Believe:	*Your Affirmation Is:*
I am afraid of sex.	*It is safe for me to explore my sexuality.*
Sex is dirty.	*Sex is tender, loving and joyful.*
Genitals frighten me.	*Genitals are normal and natural and beautiful. I don't get what I want. I am always fulfilled and satisfied sexually.*
I am the wrong size or shape.	*My genitals are perfect for me.*
I am ashamed of my sexuality.	*I go beyond limiting beliefs and accept myself totally.*
I can't ask for what I want.	*I express my desires with joy and freedom.*
God doesn't want me to be sexual.	*God created and approves of my sexuality.*
My partner won't like my body.	*My partner reflects the love I have for my body.*
I'm afraid of disease.	*I am divinely protected and guided.*
I'm not good enough.	*I love myself and my sexuality. I am at peace.*
Sex is painful.	*I am gentle with my body and so is my partner.*

"I give myself permission to enjoy my body."

POWER POINTS

1. We are each responsible for our experiences.

2. Every thought we think is creating our future.

3. Everyone is dealing with the damaging patterns of resentment, criticism, guilt, and self-hatred.

4. These are only thoughts and thoughts can be changed.

5. We need to release the past and forgive everyone, including ourselves.

6. Self-approval and self-acceptance in the "now" are the keys to positive changes.

7. The point of power is always in the present moment.

14

LOVE AND INTIMACY

"Love surrounds me. I am loving, loveable, and loved."

Love and Intimacy Checklist

☐ I'm afraid of rejection.
☐ Love never lasts.
☐ I feel trapped.
☐ Love scares me.
☐ I have to do everything *their* way.
☐ If I take care of myself, they will leave me.
☐ I'm jealous.
☐ I can't be myself.
☐ I am not good enough.
☐ I don't want a marriage like my parents had.
☐ I don't know how to love.
☐ I can't say no to someone I love.
☐ Everybody leaves me.

How many of these sound like you? You may need to dissolve the love and intimacy fears.

How did you experience love as a child? In your family was love expressed through fighting, yelling, crying, door-slamming, manipulation, control, silence, or revenge? If it was, then you will seek out similar experiences as an adult. You will find the people who will reinforce those ideas. If, as a child, you looked for love and found pain, then as an adult you will find pain instead of love until you release your old family pattern.

1. How did your last relationship end?

_____

_____

_____

_____

2. How did the one before that end?

_____

_____

_____

_____

Perhaps all of your relationships ended as a result of your partner leaving you. The need in you to be left could come from a family divorce, a parent withdrawing from you because you weren't what they wanted you to be, or a death in the family.

To change the pattern, you need to forgive your parent AND understand that you don't have to repeat this old behavior. You free them and yourself.

For every habit or pattern we repeat over and over again, there is a NEED WITHIN US for such repetition. The need corresponds to some belief that we have. If there was no need, we would not have to have it, do it, or be it. Self-criticism does not break the pattern: letting go of the need does.

MIRROR WORK

Using your mirror, look into your eyes, breathe, and say: "I am willing to release the need for relationships that do not nourish and support me."

Say this five times in the mirror; each time you say it, give it more meaning. Think of some of your relationships as you say it.

EXERCISE: *Your Relationships*

In the space below, answer the following questions as best you can.

1. What did you learn about love as a child?

_____

_____

_____

_____

2. Did you ever have a boss who was "just like" one of your parents? How?

_____

_____

_____

_____

3. Is your partner/spouse like one of your parents? How?

_____

_____

_____

_____

4. How were they alike?

_____

_____

_____

_____

5. What would you have to forgive in order to change this pattern?

_____

_____

_____

_____

6. From your new understanding, what would you like your relationship to be like?

_____

_____

_____

_____

Your old thoughts and beliefs continue to form your experiences until you let them go. Your future thoughts have not been formed, and you do not know what they will be. Your current thought, the one you are thinking right now, is totally under your control.

We are the only ones who choose our thoughts. We may habitually think the same thought over and over so that it does not seem as if we are choosing the thought. But, we did make the original choice. We can refuse to think certain thoughts. How often have you refused to think a positive thought about yourself? You can also refuse to think a negative thought about yourself. It just takes practice.

EXERCISE: *Love and Intimacy*

Let's examine these beliefs. Answer each of the questions below. After each answer write a positive affirmation (in the present tense) to replace the old belief.

1. Do I feel worthy to have an intimate relationship?

Example:
No. Another person would run if they really knew me.

YOUR EXAMPLE:

_____

_____

_____

_____

Sample Affirmation:
I am lovable and worth knowing.

YOUR AFFIRMATION:

_____

_____

_____

_____

2. **Am I afraid to love?**

Example:
Yes—I'm afraid that they won't be faithful.

YOUR EXAMPLE:

_____

_____

_____

_____

Sample Affirmation:
I am always secure in love.

YOUR AFFIRMATION:

_____

_____

_____

_____

3. What am I "getting" from this belief?

Example:
I don't let romance in my life.

YOUR EXAMPLE:

_____

_____

_____

_____

Sample Affirmation:
It is safe for me to open my heart to let love in.

YOUR AFFIRMATION:

_____

_____

_____

_____

4. What do I fear would happen if I let go of this belief?

Example:
I would be taken advantage of and be hurt.

YOUR EXAMPLE:

_____

_____

_____

_____

Sample Affirmation:
It is safe for me to share my innermost self with others.

YOUR AFFIRMATION:

_____

_____

_____

_____

EXERCISE: *Your Critical Self*

Criticism breaks down the inner spirit, and never changes a thing. Praise builds up the spirit and can bring positive changes. Write down two ways in which you criticize yourself in the area of love and intimacy. Perhaps you are not able to tell people how you feel, or what you need. Maybe you have an fear of relationships, or attract partners that will hurt you.

Then, think of a way in which you have not been acting out this behavior.

Examples:

I criticize myself for: *choosing people who are not able to give me what I need.*

I praise myself for: *telling someone that I liked them. It scared me, yet I did it anyway.*

1. **I criticize myself for:**

_____

_____

_____

_____

I praise myself for:

_____

_____

_____

_____

2. I criticize myself for:

_____

_____

_____

I praise myself for:

_____

_____

_____

_____

Congratulations! You have just begun to break another old habit! You are learning to praise yourself—in this moment. And the point of power is always in the present moment.

Review the checklist of negative beliefs on the next page, taken from page 145, and find the corresponding affirmations next to them. Make these affirmations part of your daily routine. Say them often in the car, at work, or any time you feel your negative beliefs surfacing.

If You Believe:	Your Affirmation Is:
I am afraid of rejection.	*I love and accept myself and I am safe.*
Love never lasts for me.	*Love is eternal.*
I feel trapped.	*Love makes me feel free.*
Love scares me.	*It is safe for me to be in love.*
I have to do everything *their* way.	*We are always equal partners.*
If I take care of myself, they will leave me.	*We each take care of ourselves.*
I can't be myself.	*People love me when I am myself.*
I'm not good enough.	*I am worthy of love.*
I don't want a marriage like my parents had.	*I go beyond my parents' limitations.*
I don't know how to love.	*Loving myself and others gets easier every day.*
I'll get hurt.	*The more I love, the safer I am.*
I can't say no to someone I love.	*My partner and I respect each other's decisions.*
Everybody leaves me.	*I now create a long-lasting, loving relationship.*

"I give myself permission to experience intimate love."

POWER POINTS

1. We are each responsible for our experiences.

2. Every thought we think is creating our future.

3. Everyone is dealing with the damaging patterns of resentment, criticism, guilt, and self-hatred.

4. These are only thoughts and thoughts can be changed.

5. We need to release the past and forgive everyone, including ourselves.

6. Self-approval and self-acceptance in the "now" are the keys to positive changes.

7. The point of power is always in the present moment.

PART III

YOUR NEW LIFE

YOUR NEW PICTURE

"I see myself in a new light."

With your nondominant hand (the hand you don't usually use) draw a new picture of yourself. Either use crayons or pens. Sit quietly. Close your eyes. Breathe. Center yourself.

Who are you?

Why are you here?

What have you come here to learn?

What have you come here to teach?

What has changed?

PICTURE YOURSELF HERE

WHAT MAKES ME HAPPY?

"I recognize that I am the source of my happiness."
We have explored so many areas of our lives. We have uncovered negative patterns and beliefs. We have relinquished old baggage. We feel freer and lighter. We are open and receptive to good. So the next question is: What would make you happy? This is not time to talk about what you don't want. This is a time to be very clear about what you do want in your life. List everything that you can think of. Cover all the areas of your life. List at least 50 things.

1. _____

2. _____

3. _____

4. _____

5. _____

6. _____

7. _____

8. _____

9. _____

10. _____

11. _____

12. _____

13. _____

14. _____

15. _____

16. _____

17. _____

18. _____

19. _____

20. _____

21. _____

22. _____

23. _____

24. _____

25. _____

26. _____

27. _____

28. _____

29. _____

30. _____

31. _____

32. _____

33. _____

34. _____

35. _____

36. _____

37. _____

38. _____

39. _____

40. _____

41. _____

42. _____

43. _____

44. _____

45. _____

46. _____

47. _____

48. _____

49. _____

50. _____

Now create a positive affirmation for each item. Be aware that anyone who has done as much work as you have in order to change, deserves to have a wonderful new world.

1. _____

2. _____

3. _____

4. _____

5. _____

6. _____

7. _____

8. _____

9. _____

10. _____

11. _____

12. _____

13. _____

14. _____

15. _____

16. _____

17. _____
18. _____
19. _____
20. _____
21. _____
22. _____
23. _____
24. _____
25. _____
26. _____
27. _____
28. _____
29. _____
30. _____
31. _____
32. _____
33. _____
34. _____
35. _____
36. _____
37. _____
38. _____
39. _____
40. _____
41. _____

42. _____

43. _____

44. _____

45. _____

46. _____

47. _____

48. _____

49. _____

50. _____

It is exciting to have wonderful people, places, and things in our lives. However, we must be clear that these things do not "make us happy." Only *we* can "make us happy." Only we can think the thoughts that can create peace and joy. Never give power to an outside person or source. Make yourself happy, and all good will flow to you in great abundance.

MIRROR WORK

Look into the mirror. Breathe. Smile. Say, "I deserve to have a wonderful life." Breathe again. " I deserve everything on my list." Breathe. "I deserve and accept all good in my life." Breathe. "I am a loving, worthwhile person, and I love myself." Breathe. "All is well in my world."

YOUR NEW STORY

"I see myself in a new light."

Now that you have a list of all the items you would like to have in your life—people, places, and things that could contribute to your happiness, let's put them into a story. Write as much or as little as you wish.

I, _____, now have a wonderful life. . .

_____

_____

_____

_____

_____

_____

_____

_____

_____

_____

_____

_____

_____

_____

_____

_____

_____

_____

_____

_____

VISUALIZATION

Now that you have written your new story, see yourself living it. What does you new life feel like? What do you look like as you grow older? See your harmonious relationships. Breathe in your newfound freedom and happiness.

RELAXATION AND MEDITATION

Relaxation is essential to the healing process. It is hard to allow the healing energies to flow within us if we are tense and frightened. Dr. Bernie Siegel said, "The physical benefits of meditation have been well documented. It tends to lower or normalize blood pressure, pulse rate, and the level of stress hormones in the blood. Its benefits are also multiplied when combined with regular exercise. In short, it reduces wear and tear on both body and mind, helping people live better and longer."

It only takes a moment or two, several times a day, to allow the body to let go and relax. At any moment, you can close your eyes and take two or three deep breaths and release whatever tension you may be carrying. If you have more time, sit or lie quietly, and talk your body into complete relaxation. Say silently to yourself, "My toes are relaxing, my feet are relaxing, my ankles are letting go," etc., working all the way up and down your body, or you may begin with you head and work down.

At the end of this simple exercise, you will be peaceful and calm for a while. Repeating this often can create a peaceful state within you, most of the time. This is a very positive, physical meditation that you can do anywhere.

As a society, we have made meditation into something mysterious and difficult to achieve. Yet meditation is one of the oldest and simplest processes we can do. Yes, we can make it complicated, with specialized breathing and ritualized mantras. Those meditations are fine for advanced students. Still, everyone can meditate now; it is easy to do.

All we have to do is to sit or lie quietly, close our eyes, and take a few deep breaths. The body will automatically relax; we don't have to do anything to force it. We can repeat the words "healing" or "peace" or "love" or anything that is meaningful to us. We could even say, "I love myself." We can ask silently, "What is it I need to know?" Or "I am willing to learn." Then just be there quietly.

Answers may come immediately or in a day or two. Don't feel rushed. Allow things to happen. Remember that it is the nature of the mind to think; you will never completely rid yourself of dashing thoughts. Allow them to flow through. You might notice, "Oh, now I am thinking fear thoughts or anger thoughts or disaster thoughts or whatever." Don't give these thoughts importance; just let them pass through like soft clouds in a summer sky.

Some say that uncrossing your legs and arms and sitting upright with a straight spine, will improve the quality of the meditation. Maybe so. Do it if you can. What is important is to meditate on a regular basis. The practice of meditation is cumulative: the more regularly you do it, the more your body and mind responds to the benefits of relaxation, and the quicker you may get your answers.

Another easy method of meditation is to simply count your breaths as you sit quietly with your eyes closed. Count one on the inhale, two on the exhale, three on the inhale, and so on, counting your breath from one to ten. When you exhale on ten, just begin again at one. If your mind wanders and you find yourself counting up to eighteen or thirty, merely bring yourself back to one. If you find your mind fretting about your doctor or your job or about doing a shopping list, simply bring yourself back to the count of one.

You cannot meditate incorrectly. Any starting point is perfect for you. You can find books that will teach you several methods. You may go to a class that will give you the experience of meditating with others. Begin anywhere. Allow it to become a habit.

If you are new to meditation, I would suggest that you begin with only five minutes at a time. People who immediately do twenty or thirty minutes can get bored and skip it entirely. Five minutes once or twice a day is a good beginning. If you can do it at the same time every day, the body begins to look forward to it. Meditation gives you small periods of rest that are beneficial to the healing of your emotions and body.

You see, we all have tremendous wisdom within us. Inside of us lie all the answers to all the questions we shall ever ask. You have no idea how wise you are. You can take care of yourself. You do have the answers you need. Get connected. You will feel safer and more powerful.

Know that my support is always with you. I love you.

CLOSING TREATMENT

The past is over and done. It has gone back to the nothingness from whence it came. I am free. I have a new sense of pride and self-worth. I am confident in my abilities to love and support myself. I have learned that I am capable of positive growth and change. I am strong. I am united with all of life. I am one with the Universal power and intelligence. Divine wisdom leads me and guides me every step of the way. I am safe and secure as I move forward to my highest good. I do this with ease and with joy. I am a new person, living in a world of my choosing. I am deeply grateful for all that I have and for all that I am. I am blessed and prosperous in every way. All is well in my world.

Suggested Reading

Bach, Richard, *Illusions* (New York: Dell
    Publishing, 1977).
Bailes, Fredrick, *Your Mind Can Heal You*
    (Marina Del Rey, CA: De Vorss & Co., 1941).
Bartholomew, *I Come As A Brother* (Taos, NM:
    High Mesa Press, 1986).
Beattie, Melody, *Codependent No More* (San
    Francisco, CA: Harper and Row, 1987).
Coit, Lee, *Listening* (Wildomar, CA: Las Brisas
    Retreat Center, 1985).
Cousins, Norman, *Anatomy of An Illness* (New
    York: Bantam Books, 1981).
Fox, Emmett, *Power Through Constructive
    Thinking* (San Francisco: Harper & Row,
    1968).
Gawain, Shakti, *Creative Visualization* (Mill
    Valley, CA: Whatever Publishing, 1978).
_____. *Living in the Light* (Mill Valley,
    CA: Whatever Publishing, 1986).
Gordon, Richard, *Your Healing Hands* (Berkeley,
    CA: Wingbow Press, 1978).
Harrison, John, M.D., *Love Your Disease* (Santa
    Monica, CA: Hay House, Inc., 1989).

Hay, Louise L., *You Can Heal Your Life* (Santa Monica, CA: Hay House, Inc., 1984).

——————. *Love Your Body* (Santa Monica, CA: Hay House, Inc., 1987).

——————. *Heal Your Body* (Santa Monica, CA: Hay House, Inc., 1982).

Holmes, Ernest, and Willis H. Kinnear, *A New Design For Living* (New York: Prentice Hall, 1987).

Jampolsky, Gerald, *Love Is Letting Go of Fear* (Millbrae, CA: Celestial Arts, 1979).

Jeffers, Susan, Ph.D., *Feel the Fear and Do It Anyway* (New York: Ballantine Books, 1987).

Johnson, Elizabeth A., *As Someone Dies* (Santa Monica, CA: Hay House, Inc., 1987).

Levine, Stephen, *Who Dies? An Investigation of Conscious Living and Dying* (New York: Doubleday & Co., 1982).

MacLaine, Shirley, *Out On a Limb* (New York: Bantam Books, 1983).

Moody, Raymond A., M.D., *Life After Life* (New York: Bantam Books, 1975).

Murphy, Joseph, *The Power of Your Subconscious Mind* (New York: Bantam Books, 1982).

Norwood, Robin, *Women Who Love Too Much* (New York: Pocket Books, 1985).

Pollard, John K., *Self Parenting* (Malibu, CA: Generic Human Studies Publishing, 1987).

Rodegast, Pat, and Judith Stanton, *Emmanuel's Book* (New York: Bantam Books, 1985).

Scheid, Robert, *Beyond the Love Game* (Berkeley, CA: Celestial Arts, 1980).

Seigel, Bernie, M.D., *Love, Medicine and Miracles* (New York: Harper & Row, 1986)

Serinus, Jason, ed., *Psychoimmunity and the Healing Process* (Berkeley, CA: Celestial Arts, 1986).

Shin, Florence Scovel, *The Game of Life and How to Play It* (Marina Del Rey, CA: De Vorss & Co., 1940).

Simonton, Carl, M.D., *Getting Well Again* (New York: Bantam Books, 1980).

Wilde, Stuart, *Miracles* (Taos, NM: White Dove International, Inc., 1983).